HEALING
OUTSIDE
the MARGINS

HEALING OUTSIDE the MARGINS

the Survivor's Guide to Integrative Cancer Care

Carole O'Toole

with Carolyn B. Hendricks, M.D.
Medical Advisor

LifeLine
Press®

Washington, D.C.

First Paperback Edition, 2003
Library of Congress Cataloging-in-Publication Data

O'Toole, Carole.
  Healing outside the margins: a survivor's guide to integrative
cancer care / Carole O'Toole, with Carolyn B. Hendricks.
    p. cm.
  ISBN 0-89526-193-6
1. Cancer--Alternative treatment--Popular works. I. Title.
  RC271.A62 087 2002
  616.99'406--dc21

2002000958

Published in the United States by
LifeLine Press
A Regnery Publishing Company
One Massachusetts Avenue, NW
Washington, DC 20001

Visit us at www.lifelinepress.com

Distributed to the trade by
National Book Network
4720-A Boston Way
Lanham, MD 20706

Printed on acid-free paper
Manufactured in the United States of America
Jacket design: Amy Cade
Design: Marja Walker
Author photo: Shane McCarthy, Dublin, Ireland
10 9 8 7 6 5 4 3 2 1

Books are available in quantity for promotional or premium use. Write to Director of Special Sales, Regnery Publishing, Inc., One Massachusetts Avenue, NW, Washington, DC 20001, for information on discounts and terms or call (202) 216-0600.

The information contained in this book is not intended as a substitute for medical counseling and care. All matters pertaining to your physical health should be supervised by a health care professional.

You've flapped and fluttered against limits
long enough.

You've been a bird without wings in a house
without doors or windows.

Compassion builds a door
Restlessness cuts a key

Ask!

Step off proudly into sunlight,
not looking back.

—Rumi

To Jeffrey Zitelman
and
Kiera Elizabeth O'Toole Zitelman

For holding open your hearts for me
And showing me the way back.

You are my true north.

ACKNOWLEDGMENTS

From my view, there isn't enough gratitude shared in life. It is a gift when received and an honor to express. Alice O'Toole, who brought me far in life so I could handle the rest, taught me so much about thankfulness. Being my mother, she also instilled in me the necessity of writing thank you notes . . . which is actually how this book began. It started as my way of thanking all the incredible healers who worked with me and the people living with cancer who have crossed my path. But the experience of writing this book has widened the circle: as with my illness, the Universe gave me more help, talent, and encouragement than I could have ever thought to ask for.

I don't believe I can ever adequately express my appreciation for Dr. Carolyn Hendricks, my oncologist and medical advisor to this book. During my illness, I was so fortunate to have benefited from her incredible skill as a physician, and was blessed by her devotion and friendship as well. She is a rare find, and I continue to be graced with her wisdom and generosity on this project. Her energy, optimism, and support have been a healing light, and I consider her my goddess.

Rick Steinberg, M.D., shared his experience as a physician, complementary practitioner, and cancer survivor, and much of his time in helping to make the book a reality. He wrote the original version of Chapter 2, helped in the selection of modalities, and conducted some of the practitioner and survivor interviews. My thanks to him for his many contributions and sound advice. Thanks also to Matt Hoffman and Rebecca Perl for their research and contributions to the modalities. Their talents made the difference.

I would like to acknowledge all of the talented healers who participated in interviews. As much as the book was hard work, meeting you was an unexpected joy. I am so grateful for your words as well as your prayers and encouragement, and honored to have your work reflected here. Special thanks go to the following individuals for their valuable assistance: Dr. Lisa Chun, Dr. Harold Goodman, Dr. Robert Heffron, Dr. Andrea Sullivan, Dr. Lillian Rosenbaum, Bonnie Sobel, Jill Cahn, Peggy Li, Susan Drobis, Tara Brach, Irene Morelli, Maureen McCracken, Betty Caldwell, Dr. Irv Rosenberg, Dr. Kumuda Reddy, Judy Nelson Siegal, Dr. Marc Smith, Lisa Patterson, Joan Nelson, Sharon Benoliel, Sue Greer, Bill Short, Lynn Rosen, and Ron Murray.

My appreciation extends to Dana Laake, who was invaluable in providing sound advice on nutrition, and Gary Sandman, who made me look good on paper *and* film. I am grateful to Jackie Wootton, for her sage advice and enthusiasm, and for the generosity of the Alternative Medicine Foundation, for sharing many of the resources that appear in the Appendix. I wish to gratefully acknowledge Meniscus Educational Institute as well, for allowing me to include in this book portions of material I had originally written for *Innovations in Breast Cancer Care.*

My deepest gratitude to Mary Lee Esty and Sabine Gnesdiloff—two of my treasures I found during my illness—for their advice and inspiration during the writing of this book. I have healed as much from their friendship as from their healing practice.

My gratitude also extends to the people who have faced cancer and who so freely opened their hearts and shared their wisdom, pain, and triumph with me: the focus group participants, clients of healers interviewed for the book, and especially Sue Perrine, Susan Holloran, Katherine Anthony, and Ellen Grayson. Their voices make the book more alive and meaningful, and I am most thankful for their "passing it on."

I am very thankful to three extremely creative women: Maggie Bedrossian and Lynne Waymon who, as authors, saw the spark in my idea for this book and ignited it; and Joan Wangler, a fellow writer and Coach Extraordinaire, whose coaching from the heart fanned the flame. As friends, all three have nourished the book's growth along with my own.

The book would have been abandoned long ago if it hadn't been for two true-blue friends, Dottie Cornwell and Janice Fein Dean. Dottie's infusions of humor and shuttles to medical treatments kept me sane eight years ago, and she came through again by helping me with many tasks on this book that would have driven anyone mad. Her friendship is a gift for which I will be forever grateful. Janice was a friend first before I discovered her talent as an editor. With insight and infinite patience, she gently guided me through the anguish of rewrites and made this book shine. She is truly a treasure.

Elaine Callinan and Ann Norfolk offered me unconditional support throughout the writing of this book. Elaine's critiques, research, late-night discussions on healing, and faith in this book sustained and nurtured me. This book would not be in your hands if not for her. Ann generously gave her wisdom and loving energy to numerous reviews of chapters, concepts and ideas, and tirelessly helped to birth this book. She continues to be my guide and port in *any* storm. I am in awe of both of them.

Many others were instrumental in moving the book along, and I cannot thank you enough: Andrea Newmark, for her persistent research on the appendix and modalities; Bobbi Brady, for interview assistance and focus group preparations; Mary Beth O'Toole, for interviewing clients and worrying right along with me; and Rachel Ingold, who came to the rescue in the eleventh hour. Marc Heyison and Steve Peck, co-founders of Men Against Breast Cancer, give new meaning to the term caregiver. They are angels incarnate. And my thanks to family and friends who provided retreats on both sides of the Atlantic, helping to restore my spirits and creativity when both lagged: Gaylen and Tom Camera, Alice Hogan and Marty Whyte, and Martha, Brendan, and Dominick Roche.

Turning ideas and words into such a beautiful book is an art. I am honored and deeply grateful that the following incredibly talented people made it happen: Nina Graybill, my agent, who allowed me the sheer luxury of being able to say those words, "my agent," and for teaching me a thing or two! The outstanding people at LifeLine Press: Marji Ross, for seeing beyond my backyard before I did and taking a chance on me; Mike Ward, for his patience, humor, and creative vision; Lauren Lawson and John Lalor, for making me look *really* good and pushing the book with a passion; Brian Robertson, for his calm demeanor as much as his editorial skills; and to the sweetest editor, Molly Mullen, whom I wish I had met a *lot* sooner. She got it from day one and made my initiation to publishing such a pleasant one. All of them have my admiration and appreciation for making it look so easy.

Finally, I dearly hope my husband Jeff and daughter Kiera know the depth of my gratitude for their devotion and encouragement. I am so thankful for their love and patience, and all the many ways they supported me during the seemingly endless time it took to write this book. You are my heroes; you gave me my life again. I thank God for bringing you to me.

And many people I loved that have left this life continue to send me love and guidance that have carried me through from the moment I realized I needed to write this book. I am blessed by their presence, as I continue to be blessed by God, whose mercy, grace, and guidance brought me to this place in my life. By your love I have been healed.

I am one lucky woman.

CONTENTS

AN IMPORTANT NOTE TO THE READER

One of the main messages of this book is that you more actively participate in your healing. This message should not be misinterpreted to mean you are solely responsible for managing your health care when dealing with cancer. Rather, I encourage you to learn about your illness and your options—both conventional and complementary—and discuss them with the physician you have selected to coordinate your care. Seek second opinions from physicians and other qualified health professionals when you feel you need to. And keep your resources updated: stay informed of progress made and new opportunities in both treatment areas.

Complementary therapies are valued largely for their role in maintaining general health and well-being, assisting in the healing process, and improving the quality of life. No statement in this book should be interpreted as a claim for a cure; the benefits that are cited are still mostly anecdotal, yet many are substantiated by peer-reviewed research. While there are often specific benefits attributed to certain therapies that can be very powerful assets in healing from cancer, they are not recommended here as primary or sole treatment when dealing with a life-threatening illness.

Please respect your current health circumstances and however your body is coping with them. Some complementary treatments may pose a certain level of risk, and certain therapies may be contraindicated during active cancer treatment or for particular health conditions. Please act wisely and take care in seeking out complementary therapy within the context of your limitations and/or sensitivities. As you will see, there are different approaches within modalities and among practitioners, so please keep in mind that individual experiences with each of these modalities and their practitioners may vary.

The inclusion of specific practitioners, organizations, and modalities in the book should not be interpreted as endorsements for these individuals, treatments, or organizations. This book should serve as a guide to, and not a substitute for, good holistic medical care.

It is important to note here that self-treatment with herbs and/or natural supplements is not advised. The quality and source of the herbs may not always be reliable, and possible side effects and—even more important—drug/herb interactions can put your health at risk.

In seeking complementary care, always do so under the full knowledge and guidance of your allopathic physician, who is familiar with your unique situation. If she or he is unfamiliar with complementary medicine, find a competent licensed health care practitioner or complementary practitioner who can help coordinate care with your physician and you. Involve your entire health care team: consult with both your complementary and conventional medical practitioners before receiving or resuming complementary treatment.

PART I

Moving toward
integrative cancer care

YOU MUST BE JOKING

PLAN *(plan), n., v., planned, planning—n. 1. an intended agenda. v. 2. to contemplate an intention. n. 3. a promise or gift you give to yourself.*

I t's been said that the best way to make God laugh is to make plans. With cancer, it's as if the forces of the universe have laughed at our tidy life plans and ambitions, torn them up, and scattered them to the winds. Why plan at all? Nothing makes sense any more. We no longer feel on track, in the flow of what we always assumed we were in charge of: our lives. The predictability of life's rhythm has disappeared overnight, in the blinking of an eye. We feel at the mercy of forces beyond our power to affect. Indeed, many people think it's a sure-fire bet that God is laughing if you're making plans while dealing with this disease.

Making a conscious decision to develop a personal plan for healing in the face of cancer is no laughing matter, however. Instead, it is a serious commitment to become more aligned with yourself as you begin to heal from a terrifying illness. In this context, it doesn't really matter whether your plan is ever fully realized, for healing isn't the sole outcome; it is the process as well. As you heal, you prepare yourself for further growth, expansion, and experience. It is the intention you put forth to heal as a whole person that puts you in the position to develop a healing plan.

The word "plan" is such a basic word that describes a wondrous process, and it takes on a whole new meaning in the context of cancer. I struggled long and hard with how to define "plan" for this book. It's so easy simply to adopt the medical terminology associated with complementary care, summing up your intentions and actions related to healing from cancer with the phrase "integrated treatment plan." But that didn't sit well with me, because it only gives part of the picture. It connotes a proven methodology, controlled action, and predictable results. In reality, the only certainty of an integrated treatment plan for complementary cancer care is your intention to get well. The rest unfolds under its own power and within its own time frame. You are "in charge" in the sense that you are willing to open the next door rather than have it opened for you; to look around the next corner rather than being shown it. But precisely what lies there for you—what you need to heal—remains to be discovered.

All you have when you begin looking into complementary treatments is a promise to yourself to be open to your healing and to the process by which it will be made known to you. And that's really all you need. You needn't possess a highly developed intuitive sense, nor sharp analytical skills. No proven method, sophisticated tools, or complicated procedures are necessary. Your intent is what's most important. For from that intention come amazing and unexpected gifts that are yours for the asking. The gifts I received from my healing plan—my promise to myself—extended far beyond my cancer experience. I hope some of these gifts will reach you through what you are about to read. For it is this definition of "plan" as a promise or a gift to yourself that inspired the writing of this book.

You could say that this book has a split personality. My motivation for writing it is to encourage and inspire you to get more involved in your healing from cancer, to create and realize your promise. But I know how difficult it is to get started—and to keep going. In truth, a part of this healing process *does* fit the first definition of "plan" used here. There *are* some procedures you can decide on in advance, even when you feel that nothing is certain. I want to share those with you as well. *Healing Outside the Margins,* then, is part inspirational and part instructional, offering as it does some gentle structure to a highly individual, personal process.

The responsibility for selecting complementary therapies while facing such a serious illness can be daunting. The variety and combinations of different complementary treatments are endless. Whereas some complementary therapies—such as acupuncture and yoga—have been used successfully for hundreds, even thousands, of years, others seem to spring up overnight on a regular basis, offering even more possibilities. Which is safe? Which is effective? How can you be sure of the integrity and skill of complementary treatment providers? These questions, of course, loom even larger when your life might be at stake.

Healing Outside the Margins provides a method of sorting through the enormous range of complementary treatment possibilities. In doing so, I hope it will ease your way toward fulfilling your promise. This framework provides you with clear steps that can help you create order and begin your search. Having these steps in place also gives you the comfort of having a structure to lean on when facing new choices.

Developing your integrated treatment plan can be a transforming and exhilarating experience. Out of chaos and confusion can come revelation and empowerment. Forging your own way, discovering exactly what *you* need to heal, and managing your own care is an incredibly profound experience. Just making the decision to explore complementary therapies opens you up to two very powerful healing forces:

The sheer will to participate actively in your healing gives you power, which you learn to use, and the incredible resources of the wonderful healers who are available and willing to work with you on any aspects of healing that you choose.

What is an integrated treatment plan? I define it as the process of seeking whatever you feel is necessary for healing from both conventional (allopathic) and complementary modalities. It can also refer to combining complementary therapies alone, if conventional medicine is not an option. The selected treatments are used together to support the patient optimally on all levels—physical, mental, emotional, and spiritual—throughout the disease and recovery process.

I have selected the term "complementary therapy" over "alternative medicine" throughout the book because I believe the former best supports the concept of integrative treatment. "Complementary" refers to an array of treatments outside the mainstream of conventional Western medicine that can be used to enhance, improve, and support a person's health and well-being. To me, the word "alternative" has a negative connotation, implying both a choice between two treatment options—rejecting one for another—as well as going *against* conventional methods. The term "complementary" seeks to be inclusive—whether the form selected is used as an adjunct to allopathic medicine or in combination with other unconventional treatments. Regardless of how the modality is applied, "complementary" suggests supporting an individual's natural ability to heal.

Healing Outside the Margins is not a rose-colored endorsement of complementary therapy. I welcomed and valued all of my allopathic care, and would recommend that all patients seek out the best conventional treatment they can find for themselves. But at the same time, I saw the value of complementary therapy in meeting certain needs of cancer patients that allopathic medicine cannot fill. I believe that *both* saved my life, and feel extremely blessed to have chosen a more integrative form of care. So while I certainly found that there were challenges in developing an integrated treatment plan, in the end my healing felt whole.

When I developed my own integrated treatment plan, I felt my way through the process. It was a gradual unfolding; in the midst of it, I had no idea where it would lead. Looking back, though, I can see that a framework developed over time, a means by which I could more confidently select various modalities and coordinate my care. Although it may feel as if you are about to jump into the abyss while exploring complementary therapies for cancer, you *will* land on your feet. That's what this book is all about: encouraging you to take a closer look at what is being offered in complementary cancer care and to make *conscious* choices about using complementary therapies in your healing that are based on love rather than fear. While each person's integrated treatment plan is created from his or her own situation and involves very personal choices, there is wisdom, comfort, and support to be gained from the experience of others. Use the blueprint offered here to develop your own healing plan as a starting point to build whatever you need. By giving you a framework you can adapt to your situation, I wish to help you make choices from a stronger, more informed place.

Healing Outside the Margins gives you the tools you need to reach decisions concerning complementary therapies: whether to use them, what to use and when, and how and where to find them. It explains the role and value of both conventional and complementary cancer therapies, demystifies complementary medicine, and gives advice on researching practitioners and modalities, assembling and communicating with your health care

team, and coordinating your care. You'll explore some of
the more popular complementary modalities used by
those of us living with cancer, and you'll be introduced to
many complementary practitioners who embody the
diversity and richness of the treatments that can be
applied to the cancer experience. Listening to these healers speak of their approaches to cancer (and hearing from
cancer survivors who have benefited from their complementary cancer care) makes what seems abstract and elusive more real and possible. It brings complementary
medicine to life, helps you to identify your needs and
desires and encourages you to find them for yourself. A
journal is also provided as a way of keeping you focused
and as a means to chart your course. Here you can record
your experience of developing your plan; later, perhaps,
others may benefit from your wisdom and guidance.

WHY THIS BOOK?

The idea for this book was born from sharing my ideas
and experiences with other survivors looking for complementary cancer care. From so many I heard the same
frustrations, concerns, hopes, and expectations that I had
felt when trying to blend conventional and complementary medicine into a healing plan. As I listened to each
person's story, my frustration grew over the isolation
each of us endures and the tremendous effort we expend
to find what might help us make ourselves whole again.
I learned so much from both those who helped me and
those I tried to help that I wanted to channel that collec-
tive energy and experience; to make it easier and less
lonely for those now facing their treatment decisions.

Throughout my illness, I received grace and guidance
in abundance whenever I stated my intentions from my
heart. That experience has touched all aspects of my life
and is now an integral part of all I do. In calling upon the

Divine for never-ending guidance and grace in developing *Healing Outside the Margins*, I'd like to share my intentions in writing this book:

In guiding you through the steps of developing an integrated treatment plan, I hope to demystify it for you, so that you will be less afraid to explore this option when faced with cancer. I can't take away the fear that cancer brings, but perhaps through this book, I can alleviate some of the helpless and hopeless feelings that are a part of dealing with the disease.

By describing readily available treatments and what they can do for cancer and including interviews with actual healers, I hope to facilitate your selections, thereby conserving your time and energy.

Finally, I hope this book will encourage you to take on as much of a role in your healing as you want (and are able) to, because ultimately you—not doctors or treatments—heal yourself. I want to help you to create your own gift, your own healing promise.

WHO IS THIS BOOK FOR?

Healing Outside the Margins can be a valuable resource for *anyone* living with cancer, regardless of where you fall on the disease spectrum: newly diagnosed, currently undergoing treatment, in recovery, or looking to prevent a recurrence. The book is appropriate for both first-time users of complementary therapy and seasoned clients now applying their knowledge of complementary care to their disease. The use of these modalities is discussed within the context of a life-threatening illness.

Because cancer affects not only the patient but also those who care about and for them, this book can serve many who are not directly battling the disease. Often, family members or friends are catalysts for exploring complementary therapy, encouraging the person facing cancer to look at all options. They may be asked to research various complementary treatments, or perhaps they are searching for ways to support their loved one who has cancer. The information herein can guide caregivers by suggesting ways to help and by offering insight about developing an integrated treatment plan. More informed support by care-givers, then, can reduce the stress involved in selecting and coordinating various therapies.

Physicians, nurses, social workers, and other health professionals will also benefit from increasing their knowledge of the applications of complementary thera-pies to cancer and of practitioners who provide such care. Many cancer patients want advice from their health care team about the reliability and availability of complemen-tary therapies in their area. It is my hope that this book can serve as a trusted resource for health professionals, raising their awareness about what their patients face in their search for complementary treatments. I hope it will also encourage them to reach out to the professional community of complementary care providers, a vital step in easing the burden for patients who have decided to coordinate their own care.

Developing an integrated treatment plan is an act of love and healing. Deciding to be more consciously involved in your cancer care and recovery is in itself life-affirming. But so much of the healing process takes place on a level deeper than we can be conscious of, revealing itself on its own terms, in its own time. In the meantime, it can be difficult to stay in the present, and not worry about the "what ifs." By giving you a structure for inte-grating complementary therapies, I hope this book will help you to move forward on your healing path. Choosing to integrate complementary therapy into your cancer care is still viewed by many as "taking the road less traveled." Let this book be a companion on that journey; may it serve as your guide as you make your treatment decisions.

PASSING IT ON . . .

Ultimately, all of my intentions in writing this book can be traced to one single desire: to give to the cancer community, which was so generous to me when I was ill. This desire was sparked by my friend Gerry. A former client of mine, he went through his cancer experience ahead of me. When I was diagnosed, he offered to serve as my mentor, as he knew only too well the loneliness of the cancer patient. Before this, we had known very little about each other on a personal level. But our previous "business only" relationship completely shifted as we shared our hopes and deepest fears. Many times during our phone conversations, I would begin to express my gratitude for his loving support. He would always stop me in midsentence and say, "Just pass it on, kid."

At Gerry's funeral, I was not surprised to hear the many eulogies in which the same words were spoken by his grieving friends and family. They talked of his boundless generosity and of trying unsuccessfully to repay him. Each time they were chided by Gerry, who reminded them that the greatest demonstration of gratitude was to share the love exchanged between them with someone else.

I hope you will open yourself to other survivors, as we have so much to give each other—things that many people never experience in their lifetime. Some will come and stay awhile, sharing stories of healing, or witnessing your story with compassion and empathy. Others will be like a blazing flash of light that takes your breath away in their ability to reach the depths of your soul with a single thought or action.

Offer them your wisdom, your humor, your pain, even

your silent knowing. There are many who walk with us or are coming along behind us. Please pass your love to them, since those who have shared the cancer experience can connect on profound levels and help each other heal.

AN INVITATION TO THE READER

As I began ruminating on the idea for this book, several writers warned me that books have a way of taking on a life of their own. Nothing could be more true. Once I began writing *Healing Outside the Margins*, my greatest challenge was finding a way to end it. During my numerous discussions with survivors and healers, I received a steady stream of requests and suggestions to include more and more modalities and practitioners. I began to see the boundaries I had set for the book expand with each recommendation. I made a conscious decision, however, that *Healing Outside the Margins* would *not* be a back-breaking tome filled with every conceivable treatment and healer. I knew that the real value of this book would be found not in the breadth of information it contained but in the depth and richness of the experienced voices that speak from its pages.

Ultimately, I selected modalities and practitioners primarily from my own backyard, as it's what I know best, to illustrate the richness of the resources that are readily available in many locations around the country. But it was clear at the same time that this book could *and should* contain available complementary modalities and practitioners recommended by survivors in other locations. *Healing Outside the Margins* could then truly be a book that "passes it on," elevating the networking that exists at the local level to an ongoing conversation among those with experience of cancer around the country. But for that to happen, I need more of you to pass on what you know.

I invite you to help make this book a living project by joining me in an interactive dialogue. A web site has been established to help readers share their integrative experience. The web site contains profiles of additional practitioners that I and other survivors have found in communities around the country, as well as tools to help you collect information from practitioners in your area. I would like your recommendations for modalities and healers you have found useful in healing from cancer, in order to expand the horizons for healing as more techniques and practitioners are shared among the cancer community. It is my hope that complementary cancer care guides specific to particular locations can be made available from the web site as readers pass along their experience and advice. The goal is to have a rich gathering place for complementary resources nationwide, recommended by cancer survivors themselves.

In short, I hope you will "pass it on": this is a way to share what you have learned in your healing with countless others, and help the community of survivors fulfill its potential in caring for and supporting each other. You can participate in our project by contacting us at:
www.healingoutsidethemargins.com

ABOUT THE TITLE . . .
Many cancer survivors live for those words "You had clean margins." *Yes!* Our surgeon contained the cancer and removed it. "Outside the margins" are words every cancer patient dreads. It means that the cancer is growing free, perhaps unable or unwilling to be tamed by medicine or miracles.

But I've found that cancer changes our view of reality, and often we can embrace what we once feared. It is possible to turn what we viewed as limitations and endings into possibilities and opportunities. In reality, life after a cancer diagnosis *is* outside the margins. It's beyond anything we've experienced. Life becomes a roller coaster on fast forward; the highs are higher and the lows are below rock bottom. We are plunged into a suspended state of chaos. Many cancer patients look for a way out. They want to get off this ride immediately, back to the safer, more predictable merry-go-round. And some actually do "return" to their future: treatment ends and they're back to work, back to relationships, their cancer only a blip on the screen.

Others experience cancer as a way to become more creative with their healing. Cancer has no rules; having seen their life explode outside the margins, these patients decide that their response needs to be outside the margins, too.

Healing is a very messy business. We have all seen the final product of physical healing: wounds close, scars form and fade. What it will look like in the end, though, no one knows. It is a different process for everyone. Healing is full of aches and pains, pushing and pulling, progress and setbacks. It's *all* out of the margins of predictability, which is what makes it such a wondrous process to experience.

Making a decision to use complementary therapy for cancer is new territory for most of us as well. Moving beyond standard medical care challenges us in ways we can't predict. There are no margins around your personal integrative treatment plan. The combinations of treatments you can select are endless.

Healing outside the margins is about challenging it all. In a sense it's about beating your cancer, not in terms of winning a competition, but in terms of using your cancer to *heal* by expanding your perceptions, priorities, and ways of dealing with life. Cancer can certainly make you see your life differently. Developing an integrated treat-

ment plan helps you *live* your life with cancer differently.
I'm hoping that before you finish this book you'll see those words "outside the margins" differently, too. And you can begin to move outside your own margins of fear to freedom, creating and using your own means of getting there.

CHAPTER 1

CREATING MY PROMISE: My Healing Plan

The process of healing from cancer is a very personal journey. For me, healing began the moment I was diagnosed in January 1994. With the words, "You have cancer," my life was suddenly simplified. In an instant, all my ambitions and dreams were swept away. My total focus became my survival and recovery.

My surgeon began to relay statistics and the specifics of my disease. I soon discovered that there's breast cancer, and then there's *breast cancer*. I had the latter. "Inflammatory breast cancer...extremely rare... advanced, stage III...most likely 18 months to live, at best." My husband doubled over, moaning at each word delivered by the doctor. I sat in stunned silence, unable to move from the weight of those words. I was thirty-eight, and had just negotiated a part-time work schedule so that I could spend more time with our two-year-old daughter. As the terrifying meaning of the grave prognosis began to filter through me, I realized that fighting cancer had just become my full-time job. I would need all of my energy— physical, emotional, and spiritual—to focus on survival. What I didn't realize at the time was how all-encompassing and complicated this fight for my life would become, consuming not only me but everyone who cared for me.

I dutifully maneuvered through those first dizzying days of tests, doctor selections, and treatment options. At times, I equated my cancer with an infestation of cockroaches. The "experts" advised me of their "battle plan": they would use the "big guns" to bomb the critters and "kill every one of 'em." They tried to assure me that when the smoke cleared, I'd still be standing and they would sweep away the debris. Well, there were many long nights when I had a hard time believing that I would still be in one piece after the "exterminators" had had their way with me. What's more, exterminators stay in business because those roaches somehow manage to return.

I began to waver over the medical advice being given, convinced I would never get through the brutal treatments planned for me. How could *anyone* survive five months of almost continuous chemotherapy using five toxic agents, a modified radical mastectomy, and six weeks of radiation? Not to mention a bone marrow transplant, which carries its own respectable mortality rate. My mantra became, "Whatever doesn't kill you makes you stronger." I hoped against hope it was true, because I knew I was about to find out. And I tried not to succumb to the feelings of fear and powerlessness that arose as the enormity of my planned treatment swept over me.

As I struggled to come to terms with what lay ahead, an unfamiliar voice—rising from somewhere inside— began to make itself heard, telling me there had to be something I could do *for* myself, rather than having everything done *to* me. I was used to being the passive patient, accustomed to receiving a reassuring diagnosis and surefire solution for whatever minor ailment plagued me. But now I was working without a net; there were no guarantees. And I was about to subject my body to some of the most grueling medical treatments in existence. I began to realize that I *myself* had to keep body and soul together through the dreaded onslaught of toxic drugs, surgeries, and radiation. But *how* to do that seemed as elusive as a miracle cure.

I'm a self-admitted (now recovering) logical, left-brained perfectionist, who prided herself on her attention to detail, scientific training, reasoning abilities, and thorough research skills. At the time of my diagnosis, I felt as though I couldn't *spell* intuition, let alone discover my own. But I rapidly realized that dealing with my cancer was going to require tapping into my intuitive side. You might as well have put me in a foreign country without a translator and wished me well.

But as I began the process of listening to this newly discovered inner voice, another message made itself known. Unlike in the past, when I had prided myself on being independent and self-sufficient, this time it became clear that I didn't need to—in fact, *couldn't*—figure it all out for myself. It was as if I could jettison this facade I had put up for so long and give myself permission to ask for help. A card that a friend sent me said: "Be bold... and mighty forces will come to your aid." As frightened as I was, this message was clean and pure and I knew it to be true. A tremendous weight seemed to have been removed, even though I knew I was facing an enormous challenge. Giving up my illusion of self-reliance and turning to others felt like a place from which I could ignore the fearful "what if" noise that surrounded me. Instead I could focus on the here and now. It was tremendously liberating to surrender to the *process* of healing and the potential it held, instead of wrestling with an outcome that only time would reveal. So while I understood that somehow I needed to become more proactive and create a way to deal with my disease that I could live with, I also knew that I wouldn't be alone in my struggle. Opening myself up to my intuition and acting on its wisdom: these were the beginnings of my gifts—my promise to myself.

Even though I had no idea how to begin, I clung to this gift of intuition, allowing it to drive my thoughts and steer my actions. The wisdom I received caused a power-ful shift in me, as I moved from the "I shoulds" to the "I wants." I welcomed its presence, for it empowered me to seek my *own* healing path, the path that would bring me back to wholeness.

I began with what I did know: that cancer hadn't con-fined itself to just my body. It had invaded my very being, and so needed to be treated holistically, with methods beyond what conventional medicine could provide. I have a healthy respect for the intelligence of cancer cells, and while I value the power of conventional medicine and the sheer physical force of its approach to cancer, I felt I would not heal completely without attending to my mind and soul as well. The power of this intuitive con-clusion pushed me to investigate whatever else might be "out there" for cancer patients — the so-called alterna-tive or complementary treatments — in hopes that some-where I would find something to help the healing, ease the emotional pain, or give me a brief moment of peace.

Like most, when I started my exploration of comple-mentary medicine, I had no idea what to do or where to look. I didn't set out to build an elaborate treatment plan. First of all, I was so deluged with medical treatments that I barely had time to breathe. And design a plan? I had cancer, for goodness sake! What was I doing thinking about a plan? That seemed about as useful as rearranging deck chairs on the *Titanic*. But as I began my chemother-apy, I also began to investigate complementary thera-pies—very cautiously at first, for fear of compromising my medical treatment or being dismissed by my doctors or family and friends as beyond hope. My habitual, rea-soned approach to life's challenges made me uncomfort-able with the idea of using my intuition for critical health decisions. Besides, I had virtually no experience with alternative treatments and no idea how to access them.

Seeking a safe haven, I approached the new-found friends in my cancer support group; these courageous partners were far better versed than I in outsmarting our disease. I thought I was ready for anything that could offer me some support. But I certainly was not prepared for the tidal wave of tips, referrals, suggestions, and conflicting advice! Like Alice falling down the rabbit hole, I began a descent into an underground of new-age choices, ancient remedies, and newly discovered curatives from exotic places, half of whose names I couldn't even pronounce.

I spent time on the Internet, deciphering testimonies from strangers and anecdotal stories of miracle cures that usually left me feeling more isolated than inspired. Scouring bookstores, I parked myself in the health section and poured over every available resource on alternative treatments: from 800-page tomes covering everything you ever wanted to know about alternative medicine to personal success stories of conquering cancer using everything from coffee enemas to Gregorian chants. There were conspiratorial discourses on the ineptitude of conventional medicine, offering horror stories of life after conventional cancer treatment while glorifying alternative care. Some authors tried to convince me that not only was I responsible for my healing but for my disease as well! I refused to assume the guilt and tried to move on. But how would I ever slog through the mountain of information that lay before me? Which treatments were reliable? Effective? Doable?

My daily routine was totally transformed as I moved from manager, wife, and mother to cancer patient and complementary therapy researcher. My professional skills were now applied to managing my treatment schedule, researching options, and making treatment decisions. I transferred much of my parental responsibility to my husband, friends, and family, who lovingly took on extra duties and gave me the time and space I needed to explore every avenue of information.

I continued to sift through treatment claims and anecdotes, talking with strangers across the country and trying to identify reputable treatment providers. At times, I had up to six sessions weekly with various healers, sandwiched in between my daily chemotherapy appointments.

Such bounty is all well and good for those who are blessed with wellness, who have the luxury of leisure time to pursue various ways to maintain their good health. But let's face it: when dealing with cancer, that sense of security goes out the window. You are now working under the most stressful circumstances imaginable. You've lost faith in your body, perhaps your doctor; you live, sleep, eat, and breathe *time*. How much do you have? What should you do with it? You're pumped on adrenaline and exhausted from the relentless fear that wakes you in the morning and sleeps with you at night. Suddenly you find yourself talking with strangers about their acupuncturist. You camp out on bookstore and library floors, searching for any evidence of a successful alternative treatment for your type of cancer. You anxiously call yet another cancer patient who uses complementary therapies, only to find that she has used fifteen different treatments.

The evolutionary state, at the time, of complementary therapy information for cancer patients had me searching for healers largely through word of mouth, and sometimes exhaustive research. Recommendations were often hard to come by. Everyone has a doctor, but who refers you to their polarity therapist? Although I was fortunate to have a wide variety of exceptional healers in my community, I found that as a cancer patient I needed to be a voracious reader, persistent researcher, skilled networker, and intuitive decision-maker...all while undergoing treatment for a life-threatening illness.

Family and friends did help with my search for treatments, but I felt I was the only one who could determine what was ultimately right for me. I was extremely fortunate to find a medical team tolerant of my use of complementary therapies, but they could offer no assistance in my search because they either had no experience with complementary treatment or had little time or interest in expanding their knowledge.

I found I was educating my physicians on my findings, and soon became known as the resident expert on complementary treatments. I was besieged by phone calls from total strangers who were several steps behind me in their own investigations. We expressed our mutual feelings of frustration, confusion, and exhaustion from our individual quests. But regardless of our respective experiences with complementary therapy, we found that we wanted to help each other heal and to empower ourselves through this process. That in itself was a very comforting and enabling force in my life. It helped lift the burden of isolation and helplessness so pervasive among cancer patients in this situation.

Through trial and error—and a tremendous amount of hard work—I assembled an integrated treatment plan piece-by-piece, blending my intuition with my intellect. I put together a team of complementary healers who gave me excellent care and were instrumental in helping me regain my health. Between my chemotherapy sessions (and with my doctor's concurrence) I met with an acupuncturist, a polarity therapist, a yoga instructor, and an energy healer. I consulted with nutritionists, changed my diet, committed myself to a regular exercise plan, and began using supplements and herbal therapies. I learned visualization, guided imagery, autogenics, and biofeedback. I began to meditate daily. And as I started to make these changes, I felt healing taking place on many levels, and in many areas of my life.

My treatment plan certainly didn't happen overnight. I constantly assessed where I was and what I needed, shifting priorities and changing direction. My plan is *still* evolving, as I continue to discover new opportunities for growth and healing. At times, finding my way through all the complementary therapies available to me seemed as daunting as my medical treatments. But as I felt the positive changes resulting from my treatment choices, my faith began to outweigh the fatigue and frustration.

I approached my healers with not much more than an intention to survive and flourish, either without or despite my disease. I told them of my fears and lack of knowledge about their methods and outcomes for cancer patients. In return, they responded with integrity and honesty. We agreed to feel our way through the cancer together. They also shared their knowledge and experience concerning how and why people heal. At times it seemed that the actual physical disease was of little consequence, as we focused together on the various levels of healing that were taking place within me. It helped me to shift some of the power I had ceded to the cancer back to *me*.

We worked in true partnership. If one of us felt that a shift was needed in treatment, we would look for a new approach together. In some cases, we decided to end our partnership so I might move on to something else. While I sought these healers' professional expertise, they also sought mine, asking about my body and what it would require to heal. It was a tremendously empowering experience, in which I learned not only to trust myself (after my body's betrayal), but also how to direct my recovery on a multitude of levels.

Gradually my attitude changed toward the conventional treatments I was undergoing so that I could approach them with less fear and more joy for the healing they could bring. Through my integrative treatment experience, I developed a fascination for and an appreciation of the many levels at which healing must take place, and the total commitment of heart and soul that is necessary to heal from such a serious illness. By helping me to focus on the process and not the outcome, I reached a peace with my cancer that I had thought was unattainable.

As I have continued to rely on my promise to be more empowered and creative in my healing and to ask for help, I have seen that God does indeed provide whatever you need to make it happen. From that realization, I have opened myself to receive the Divine love and grace that had always been available but that I had never consciously experienced. This has brought me a truly profound sense of being deeply cared for and connected to the earth, as well as a better understanding of the miraculous power of healing.

CHAPTER 2

WHAT COMPLEMENTARY and CONVENTIONAL MEDICINE HAVE to OFFER

C oming to terms with a diagnosis of cancer demands difficult choices. We are called to set out on a life-saving search for the best resources we can find. For many, that search begins and ends with allopathic—or conventional—medicine, the predominant health care system most familiar to us. But the universe of potential cancer treatments has expanded to embrace many approaches that have been termed "alternative" or "complementary" to allopathic medicine. Cancer care increasingly means the incorporation of both complementary and conventional medicine into our treatment. Both forms of care are now valued and used by cancer patients more than ever—often for very different reasons and to produce very different outcomes.

Complementary and conventional treatments have distinct approaches to healing and different roles to play in the recovery from cancer. Together, they can be a tremendous force in our healing. I have no doubt that my medical treatments saved my life. And I am convinced that without my complementary therapies I would not have survived *and* triumphed over my illness, which forever transformed the meaning of cancer for me. But I started out in the same place that most of us do, wondering how the two forms of care could fit together and, more importantly, how to use them both wisely and well.

While cancer gave my life more drama than I could have ever wanted, it is not a glamorous disease by any stretch of the imagination. Even though I benefited from the latest in advanced medical technology, the basic approach to treating the disease had not changed; I would receive chemotherapy, surgery, and radiation, the weapons of choice for over forty years. As severe as its manifestation was, my cancer would be a chronic condition if I were lucky. In my case, the word "cure" was never mentioned.

I willingly accepted whatever was recommended by my physicians. I wouldn't rest unless I knew that I was doing everything that I could for myself medically. I was not facing a slow-growing cancer; I had a five-centimeter tumor of a cancer type that was infamous for its voracity. I needed the expertise of the best breast cancer specialists and researchers and the most medically aggressive techniques I could find to stop it in its tracks, or at least get it under control.

I was reassured that everything medically possible was being done for me, and I truly welcomed my conventional cancer care. But at the same time, I began to see that it wasn't just the disease but also the medical treatment that drew me away from my normal life. As much as I tried to resist, the sheer power of the treatments transformed me from a person—a wife, mother, sister, daughter, friend, and colleague—into a patient with advanced breast cancer. I felt that a wall was being built between my physical self and the rest of me, between my old life and whatever lay beyond my cancer. Just seeing the reaction on doctors' faces when they read my diagnosis further alienated me from my old life: with each grim look I received, I felt another stone being placed on that wall.

No one will deny how physically arduous conventional cancer treatment is. I turned to complementary treatments in part out of a desire to survive this experience with as much of "me" left as possible. Complementary therapy offered me the emotional and spiritual support I needed and physically nurtured my body through its medical ordeal.

So I used complementary therapy to redefine my cancer experience. And it often succeeded, at times in seemingly insignificant, but ultimately very powerful ways. For instance, being in isolation with "biohazard" signs posted on my hospital door only emphasized for me the gravity of my situation and my feelings of loneliness. But having my massage therapist visit me during isolation helped restore some of my energy, release tension, and reconnect me with myself and others. Practicing daily visualizations of my immune system flourishing while charting the progress of my immune system's recovery, which was posted on my hospital wall, motivated me to keep up my practice, and helped me feel that I was actively contributing to my recovery. Using complementary treatment during conventional therapy kept me more focused in the present and aware of the role I could play in my healing.

Complementary treatments gave me a broader view— an approach that focused on my total well-being. The disease I had became almost irrelevant at times. The complementary work lessened the enormity of what I faced, keeping me focused on improving my coping skills and reducing my pain and suffering in ways I could manage, rather than feeling totally dependent on drugs or medical procedures. It also helped me reestablish trust in my body. Instead of loathing my disease, I learned to love myself *with* cancer and the side effects of treatment I had to learn to live with. I came to view myself less as a victim of cancer and its medical treatment, and more as an active participant in my own healing and return to health.

Many cancer patients have found complementary medicine to be the "missing link" in recovering from cancer.

A recent study of the use of complementary medicine at a comprehensive cancer treatment center reported that a large majority of patients combine their use of complementary therapy with conventional medicine.[1] You have the opportunity to use two very different approaches to healing, both of which can be tremendous assets in your cancer care. The challenge is to build on their separate strengths and know how and when to use them individually or in combination to enhance their effectiveness. You will be best served by both kinds of treatment if you can clarify the value of each and the roles they can play.

Let's review each of these approaches, then, highlighting their strengths and weaknesses. In reading this material, I hope you can take a step back from your immediate situation and acquire a better understanding and appreciation of the ways these two approaches can contribute to healing. Then you will be better able to optimize the resources you find to create a personalized healing plan.

COMPARING APPROACHES

Probably the most fundamental difference between allopathic and complementary therapies can be found in their philosophies about health. These ideas are foundations upon which they build their approaches to disease.

Allopathic medicine defines health as the absence of disease. Its whole orientation toward health is to diagnose and suppress presenting symptoms and eliminate external pathogens that create disease. Health is then viewed as restored. Through allopathic medicine, many diseases have been diagnosed that would have been difficult to discover otherwise, and many serious, life-threatening conditions have been successfully treated.

While allopathic medicine's approach of categorizing disease and symptom complexes and treating the symptoms has been very effective, it does have its limitations. For example, conventional medicine can slow the progressive bone loss associated with osteoporosis, but that does not change the underlying causes. With cancer, conventional therapies may be able to shrink a tumor but this does not change the conditions under which the tumor grew.

Complementary medicine views health as a state of balance and well-being. The symptoms of disease are often seen as a message from a body that it is under too much stress, whether from work overload, personal relationships, emotional conflicts, environmental exposure, or other origins. Complementary medicine attempts to understand and reduce the stresses that disrupt balance in the body and cause disease. Healers believe that since the physical body reflects the mental and emotional state of a being, disease can be transformed to health through an improved state of well-being. Patients try to rebuild their health in *all* facets of their lives; they strive to live healthier lifestyles, get in touch with feelings that may impact their health, or learn how to live more fulfilling lives. This is not a "new" concept emerging from a shift in consciousness; it can be traced back to the third century B.C. teachings of Hippocrates, and was embraced in the nineteenth century by Louis Pasteur, the father of microbiology.[2]

Many complementary practitioners question whether the goal of treatment should be to eliminate symptoms if they are manifestations of the body's attempt to heal itself. If symptoms are messages from the body that its equilibrium has been disturbed, is it wise to silence the message or is it better to search for the cause of the disturbance? There is no question that when a serious crisis arises, modern medical technologies usually offer the best chance for survival in the short term—but where do we go from there? Is the same approach used to save a life an optimal—or even appropriate—choice for a chronic or less life-threatening condition? Is the elimination of symptoms really equivalent with health? For example, you might continually experience stress at work or be in a relationship in which you frequently experience hostility. These situations can cause a chronic state of sympathetic nervous system hyperactivity, straining the adrenal and thyroid glands, raising blood pressure, increasing cortisol production, and decreasing immune function. Our attempts to compensate may also include chronic muscle tension, joint pain, and decreased respiration/shallow breathing. Rather than rely solely on medical intervention to reduce the physical symptoms of stress, if we can learn instead to change the way we react to these stresses, we can change the amount of stress that our bodies experience. Modalities such as yoga, meditation, and massage reduce the impact of stress on the body without medication and allow us to recover from illness by having more of our own internal resources readily available.

Allopathic medicine is especially useful for life-threatening conditions. It is a disease-oriented system, valued generally for its laser-like method of diagnosis and often dramatic, technologically superior, scientifically defensible, and cure-driven "eradication" approach. Surgical repair of an inflamed organ, electrical stimulation of a heart that has stopped beating, or intravenous antibiotics for an infection that has spread to the bloodstream are a few of the situations that show the strength of allopathic medicine. Its practitioners must go through rigorous training and credentialing, inspiring confidence in those who use the system. It uses drugs, surgery, and other forms of treatment that have withstood rigorous scientific testing on large populations. Allopathic medicine employs advanced technologies to diagnose many diseases that are not typically found in complementary modalities. It offers the high drama, "big guns" form of treatment, particularly when it comes to acute situations.

Many people believe that allopathic medicine is the best—and sometimes only—way to get better. Unfortunately, patients are sometimes told that when allopathic medicine isn't appropriate or has nothing to offer, nothing else can be done. The power of allopathic medicine can sometimes overshadow other options that, while not as technologically sophisticated or dramatic in their immediate effects, can nonetheless contribute significantly to a person's healing.

Complementary therapies lack the measurable efficiency, the cause and effect, of the allopathic approach. They encompass a wide variety of modalities that vary in precision, proven efficacy, and consistency with regard to the level and quality of practitioner training. Concerns have been raised about whether complementary therapies can actually interfere with allopathic medical treatments or possibly be detrimental to a patient's health under certain conditions.

Complementary medicine has long been criticized for these significant shortcomings. Reproducible studies of successful treatments are only just beginning to be visible in some fields of complementary and alternative medicine. It is striking how many claims are made for products and treatments with only anecdotal reports to support them. Many complementary treatments don't have the scientific safety net of published, reproducible research to back up their claims. And while many complementary modalities require their practitioners to complete extensive training programs and meet strict requirements for credentialing and licensure, other modalities have such a broad or vague focus that measurement of efficacy is difficult, training can't be delineated, and accountability is virtually impossible to enforce.

Regardless of their acknowledged popularity, the lack of scientific proof of their efficacy and professional standards has lessened the credibility of complementary therapy for many. Because of this, critics have grouped home remedies, medical folklore, old wives' tales, and new-age fads with respected complementary modalities under the heading "alternative medicine," and dismissed the whole lot as ineffective at best and, at worst, harmful.

As with anything "new," complementary therapy continues to evolve as I write these words. With that constant change come all the concomitant confusion, inconsistency, erratic application, unqualified practitioners, lack of regulation, and misinformation associated with rapid growth. Some complementary modalities matured as professions as recently as the 1970s, such as Rolfing and therapeutic touch. Subsequent teachers and practitioners continue to redefine, refine, and expand upon the model designed by an original founder. Other modalities—such as Chinese medicine, acupuncture, tai chi, qi gong, and Ayurveda—have existed in other parts of the world for thousands of years and are in the process of being adapted to appropriate applications here in the West.

Many complementary modalities are now developing and modifying teacher-training protocols, certification, and oversight requirements; forming associations for dissemination of information among professionals and to the public; regulating the spread of concepts and techniques; and codifying standards of practice. Many are growing exponentially in numbers of practitioners, as well as in public interest and regulations.

There's no doubt that we are living in a time of rapid expansion of knowledge and professional opportunities in the field of health care. Change and growth in any aspect of life are messy. "Let the buyer beware" is a caveat well worth respecting for the foreseeable future.

THE MIND-BODY CONNECTION

The medical establishment's usual view of complementary therapies is that many of their benefits are simply placebo effects rather than the willfull power of the mind to influence the body. Yet even a study of conventional medical treatments later found to be ineffective showed that as many as 70 percent of patients still had excellent or good outcomes, demonstrating the power of the physician's belief in the treatment and the patient's belief in the physician.[3] Dr. Carl Simonton, a radiation oncologist, is known for his work with patients who have appeared to recover from untreatable cancer using visualization—a mind-body technique that involves positive mental imagery. Dr. David Spiegel's work showing that support groups double the survival rates of women with metastatic breast cancer is another example of the power of the mind-body connection.[4] Research has correlated the physiological responses of improved immune function with the experience of joy and other positive emotions. According to psychologist Pat Norris, author of *Why Me? Harnessing the Healing Power of the Human Spirit* (Walpole, Mass: Stillpoint, 1985), "Hope has a neuroendocrinological effect on the body—hope affects brain chemistry, beliefs have biological consequences." On the other end of the spectrum, depression and fear produce inflammatory proteins in the body. This aspect of healing has been traditionally ignored by allopathic medicine, but it is at the heart of many complementary therapies.

The mind-body connection and its powerful relationship to healing illustrates another fundamental difference between allopathic and complementary forms of treatment. Complementary medicine relies heavily upon inner resources, especially the tremendous healing power of the mind. Allopathic medicine primarily looks to technology and external sources of treatment to determine outcome.

In dealing with disease, allopathic medicine espouses prevention and, whenever possible, early detection. It often involves invasive tests, drugs, and uncomfortable procedures. For cancer, treatment can be aggressive; toxic systemic procedures such as chemotherapy may be used, along with irradiation and surgical removal of tumors. Sometimes experimental treatments still under investigation are recommended. The treatments are intended to separate you from your cancer through external measures performed by highly trained specialists.

Complementary therapies propose to work in a more "environmentally friendly" and ecologically balanced way, generally using less toxic treatments and less aggressive approaches to helping patients recover from illness. They support patients' innate capacity for healing, with the practitioner as guide offering expertise and support. Modalities such as acupuncture, homeopathy, ayurvedic medicine, macrobiotic diets, and body work therapies, to name a few, are holistic in nature; they tap into the patient's own resources to restore health. Complementary medicine emphasizes the use of natural substances and gentle, noninvasive therapies. It is less apt to affect the individual's physical and energetic balance with drastic side effects. This is a very attractive benefit, considering that adverse reactions from allopathic medicines are a leading cause of death in this country, according to the *Journal of the American Medical Association*.[5] (There are no comparable data for adverse reactions to complementary care.)

Besides having significant side effects, the delivery of allopathic treatments often can leave a patient feeling helpless and emotionally adrift for what can be a very frightening experience. This does not mean that patients with cancer should not take advantage of what conventional medicine has to offer. Chemotherapy, radiation, surgery, and other conventional cancer treatments save lives: this is the strength and focus of allopathic medicine. But the combination of such drastic cancer treatments, along with the compartmentalization and fragmentation of self that can be experienced during treatment, sometimes leaves patients with emotional trauma.

Complementary medicine operates in partnership with patients, often empowering them with the tools they need to begin to heal themselves. The emphasis is on encouraging the body to use its own resources to restore balance and health in mind, body, and spirit. In establishing a working partnership with complementary practitioners, patients feel they are heard and acknowledged, a need that has often gone unfulfilled in the allopathic model. A recent study of breast cancer survivors in Canada showed that while these patients appreciate the honesty and technical expertise of their physicians, their complementary practitioners were praised for their emotional support and listening skills.[6] This partnership approach to healing can help reduce the feelings of helplessness and victimization that often accompany a cancer diagnosis, and improve patient satisfaction—and perhaps even outcome—as patients are given the chance to voice their concerns and receive encouragement. Unfortunately, traditional allopathic interaction with patients, which is experienced by many as too authoritarian in its approach, does not offer an opportunity for patients to become more engaged in their health decisions and the healing process.

Thus, despite the criticisms and shortcomings, the reputation of complementary medicine has steadily improved among cancer patients as both dissatisfaction with the sterility of modern medicine and recognition of the holistic relationship of mind, body, and spirit to healing have increased. The impact of complementary modalities on the quality of life of people dealing with cancer is significant. Many kinds of treatments can be powerful in assisting the healing process and restoring patients to better health. Complementary medicine often fills the emotional and spiritual void not addressed by conventional medicine.

Many patients are looking for better balance by trying to establish a more peaceful co-existence between both forms of treatment. This has already occurred in several other countries, where medical doctors routinely prescribe alternative treatments and hospitals provide true integrative care, and where patients are offered both allopathic and traditional medicine. The differences between the two illustrate that in many ways, they are mirror images that truly complement each other as components of an integrated whole. The following chart, which contrasts commonly held perceptions about conventional and complementary care, illustrates this relationship:

COMPARISON OF CONVENTIONAL AND COMPLEMENTARY MEDICINE

	ALLOPATHIC	COMPLEMENTARY
Philosophy	Disease = absence of health	Disease = state of imbalance
Approach	Disconnect diseased part from whole (exclusive). Targets illness and symptoms; efficient and focused.	Reconnect part/system to whole (inclusive). Strengthen/improve function to deal with underlying causes and restore body/mind/spirit balance.
Intensity	Results-oriented; invasive, with higher potential for significant side effects.	Process-oriented; subtle, sometimes immeasurable, indicators of progress. Many forms considered to be gentle and generally safe. (Can also have significant side effects.)
Efficacy/ Credibility	More scientifically supportable evidence for efficacy administered by highly trained specialists. Allows access to best science and technology available.	More likely anecdotal evidence/unproven effects. Practitioners at various levels of training and accountability.
Patient Interaction	Often viewed as authoritarian in approach; patient has little autonomy.	Considered to have more nurturing approach; patient in partnership with practitioner.
Outcome	Addresses immediate, life-threatening situations. Can, in some cases, cure cancer, detect it early, prevent its spread and/or prevent recurrence. Provides relief from physical symptoms of cancer. Treatments can negatively impact quality of life.	Can improve functioning of all body systems; supports natural healing ability. Improves quality of life physically, emotionally, and spiritually. Encourages participation in own healing; reduces helplessness/victimization. Supports person to cope better with disease and effects of treatment.

Whether one is receiving palliative care (care that relieves without curing) or is fortunate enough to either be cured or experience a remission from cancer using conventional treatment, complementary therapy can still play an important role. Recovery from medical procedures can be traumatic and arduous, altering one's life in a dramatic way. Complementary therapy assists by reducing the side effects of treatment and by helping to restore body, emotions, and spirit following treatment. Complementary therapy is also increasingly valued for its contributions to palliative end-of-life care. In both circumstances, complementary therapy facilitates healing at levels other than the physical, profoundly affecting our quality of life and making us more conscious of the miraculous nature of healing.

Beginning or continuing complementary therapies after medical treatment has ended can help with the transition back into everyday life by facilitating lifestyle changes, keeping you focused on continuing your healing process, and maintaining your overall well-being. Recovery from cancer treatment doesn't end with a doctor's pronouncement. While there can be a definitive end to medical treatment, regaining your health doesn't happen instantaneously. Your use of complementary therapy can continue well beyond your medical care, for as long as you feel you are benefiting from it.

Complementary therapy offers you a wide range of resources to call upon in reintegrating yourself, and can make the experience very nurturing and positive. Allopathic treatment offers the power of scientific expertise and medical technology not found elsewhere. Complementary treatment offers a variety of process-oriented resources leading to a better understanding of yourself, while motivating you to take responsibility for your own health care, and nurturing body, psyche, and spirit. By integrating both forms of medicine into your healing plan you are combining the best resources at hand to recover from both the disease and the treatments themselves. And it will give you the best chance of reducing your susceptibility to future illness and improving your quality of life.

Now *that's* something worth looking into.

CHAPTER 3

FINDING YOUR WAY

W hen you begin to investigate complementary cancer treatments, it can feel as though you are inching your way along a long, lonely road, as Dorothy and her friends did when seeking the Wizard of Oz. It seemed to them that a powerful presence loomed ahead that could give them their heart's desire—but could just as easily end their lives. They felt their future depended on the whim of a mysterious, possibly dangerous being who seemed larger than life. But when they confronted the unknown, they found that the man behind the curtain was a benign instrument through which they could reach their goals. More importantly, they discovered their own power. Their ability to heal had been right there with them all along.

So it is with developing your integrated treatment plan. When designed with wisdom and conviction, it can be an invaluable instrument to help you discover your own healing power. But how do you move from confusion and fear to focus and commitment? What, exactly, holds us back from exploring complementary medicine?

Many of us are deterred from using this amazing resource by our ignorance of what to expect from it, or how to fit it into our lives with cancer. We can be unwilling to identify and work through our fears. Sometimes it's easier to keep something so unfamiliar shrouded in mystery. We're already facing a complex disease as we struggle with conflicting, incomplete, and changing information. If dealing with cancer feels as though you're aiming at a moving target, exploring complementary cancer therapy can feel like you're aiming at it blindfolded. In the midst of a life-threatening illness, we probably feel that we can live without even more uncertainty.

When I was unsure of what to do, I tried to take Dr. Bernie Siegel's words to heart: "In the absence of certainty, there is nothing wrong with hope." For me, complementary therapy held a strong attraction: the hope of comfort, support, and control over my disease—even the glimmer of a cure.

But just as strong were my fears. Complementary medicine had a reputation as a haven for quacks and charlatans. I faced the possibility of further harming my health or depleting the strength I needed to fight my illness. Certainly, it would require a gamble of time and money. And I anticipated a lengthy search for acceptable treatments.

At times desire and dread weighed equally on my mind when I began to investigate complementary medicine. Although many cancer survivors seem just as ambivalent, a recent survey of over 400 cancer patients receiving care from the University of Texas M.D. Anderson Cancer Center showed that 83 percent of the patients with various diagnoses acknowledged their use of at least one complementary therapy.[1]

My own experience and the observations of other survivors have shown me that choosing an integrative approach is a heroic choice. It is a courageous, conscious step toward healing, stemming from a desire to improve your quality of life and use the experience of cancer to embrace healing on *all* levels, regardless of the physical outcome. Using complementary therapy for cancer is life-affirming; after all, healing isn't only about destroying the disease with conventional medicine. It can also clear away emotional debris and awaken spiritual growth so that life's meaning is enriched and cherished even more.

Even the process of developing an integrated treatment plan can be a means of fulfillment. Through the creative experience of choosing to be more actively involved in your healing, you can reach a profound place of understanding, acceptance, and self-love. Finding what is true for you, working with healers who approach disease outside the medical model, and experiencing healing in a more complete and meaningful way can lead to a transformation of heart and mind.

Choosing complementary therapy can be a powerful act if it comes from a place of strength. That doesn't mean you will overcome all your fears or embrace every complementary treatment with confidence. Instead you gently come to an understanding that particular kinds of complementary treatments can help you toward healing, and that clarity overcomes your fear.

This chapter is meant to help you find your center—the source of your conviction—that will carry you through any reluctance you may feel in your search and bring you to what is most important to you. It's about coming to know yourself better and getting your priorities in order before embarking on your personal healing plan. I designed several exercises that I used when I was putting together my treatment plan, which we will explore together here. These exercises can help increase your comfort level in moving forward and pulling together your personal plan. We'll clarify our purpose in using complementary therapy, define our limitations and priorities, and visualize our life with (and without) complementary therapy. In addition, we will examine the roadblocks and tripwires that keep us from going forward with a personal healing plan. By working through these issues, you'll begin to see how you can incorporate complementary medicine into your life, transforming the inertia of doubt into an eagerness to explore what is available to you.

These exercises are designed to help you be more comfortable with incorporating complementary therapy into your healing regimen—to help you decide what you need in order to live life *well* with cancer and whether complementary therapy will help you to fulfill those needs. You'll then be more confident about exploring these therapies further.

Before we begin, there are a few points to be made. I recognize that many cancer survivors are even more reluctant to try conventional medicine than complementary therapy. If you fit this description, it will still be useful for you to read this chapter, since it will help you organize your selection of therapies and think about some issues surrounding complementary medicine that you may not have addressed yet. After completing these exercises, some of you may decide that complementary therapy is not appropriate, at least for now. If this is true for you, your exploration is still a success, as you have considered questions that led you to your decision; the exercises may serve you well later if you decide to revisit complementary therapy in the future. Many of the questions in this chapter can be applied to conventional care as well, helping you to approach your conventional treatment a little differently, from a stronger place. Chapter 4, Creating Your Plan, may also be of help because much of it can be applied to working with conventional health practitioners.

Reactions to these exercises vary widely. Depending on where you are in your illness, your own personality and decision-making style, and your preconceptions about complementary therapy, you may find these exercises to be relatively painless, with answers coming quite easily.

On the other hand, you may not feel you have any of the answers, and that you have, instead, become even more confused! Keep in mind that the whole process of designing an integrated treatment plan is just that: a process. It is both subjective and highly personal, revealing itself on its own terms, in its own time. Whenever uncertainty sets in—and it will—try to stay in that space of "unknowing." Giving yourself the time and space you need will reveal the answers that are right for *you*.

This chapter contains much information; it can be a lot to absorb all at once. It helps to keep in mind that you are at the beginning of a journey, not a race. So I would encourage you to take in only as much as you can at one time, to turn to it when you feel you need to, and to try to pace yourself. That way, you'll be more apt to find what you need to help you along your way.

Finally, most of us find that our goals and needs change as we arrive at new stages in our healing. Often, recognizing a new stage can be a signal to reassess priorities and expectations. Whenever you reach one of these points or just want a reality check, you may want to return to these exercises; they are meant to be a lifeline in times of uncertainty. It might be helpful to record your answers and reactions to the exercises in the book's journal. Reviewing your earlier answers can sometimes help to clarify a current dilemma or remind you of your progress.

MY OWN QUESTIONS

In my medical treatment, I was slated to receive a prescribed course of action planned by professionals. But suddenly I found that I would be in charge of my complementary treatment plan, a role I wasn't sure I could take on. All of my life, I had felt reasonably comfortable taking orders from my physician. Since cancer was so complicated, I was comforted, at first, by the thought that I had an experienced medical team who offered seasoned advice, steering me clear of potential problems. But in researching my illness, as I began to grasp the rarity and severity of it, I was left with more questions than answers about my course of medical care. Complementary therapy began to loom larger as an option. But along with that choice came a great deal of internal conflict.

The war of indecision began in my head. "The doctors sure don't seem to know where this is going to go." "What the hell—I've got cancer—why should I be afraid to try complementary therapy?" "I've got to have more of a say in this! This is my life, my body: I've got to do whatever it takes to get through this!" "Do you have any idea what you're getting into? What do you think you're doing with all this complementary stuff? How will you ever sort it all out?"

I wasn't ready to dismiss complementary therapy just because it seemed chancy and unfamiliar. But I needed to narrow it down to a more manageable size and demystify it before I could decide whether to accept it.

It seemed natural to begin by looking at complementary therapy with regard to my desired outcome. So I asked myself: What did I expect from complementary treatment?

I studied how complementary therapy was being used by other cancer survivors. It quickly became apparent that there was a wide variety of motivations. Others looked to complementary treatments to:

- alleviate or eliminate physical pain/symptoms
- reduce side effects of conventional treatments
- increase overall comfort and well-being
- reduce stress
- strengthen the immune system
- assist in recovery and adopting a healthier lifestyle
- prevent recurrence/sustain health

- improve outlook and attitude
- boost energy/lessen fatigue
- find emotional support
- feel more in control
- explore spirituality
- find a cure
- assist in/support the dying process
- find peace

I knew I wanted to live as well as I could for whatever time I had. I wanted to reduce the sense of loneliness and isolation I already felt as a cancer patient and get through my medical treatment with as much of myself intact and thriving as possible. I decided if I had to go through the pain of cancer and possibly lose my life from it, that I wanted to grow and learn from the experience, and even make peace with it. And I hoped complementary therapy might help me get to that stage.

■ EXERCISE 1: Identifying Goals

Identifying goals and examining expectations can put complementary therapy into better perspective. As you begin to personalize it, you bring it more into focus in your mind, making it a potentially significant part of your healing plan. For instance, determining that your primary goal in using complementary therapy is to reduce pain will help you focus on finding therapies commonly used in pain management. Using complementary therapy specifically to improve your attitude will, of course, cause you to take different steps.

So let's look at what *you* are asking from complementary therapy. What do you think it can offer you? What are your goals within the framework of your cancer experience?

It may help you to organize your goals within the categories of holistic healing. In other words, ask yourself:

What needs to heal within you physically? Mentally? Emotionally? Spiritually? Review the list of expectations above and see if any match yours or help you to identify others. Are you looking at complementary therapy for support during or after conventional treatment? Or as your only or primary treatment? Are you hoping it will help you live your life the way you want to? How do you think complementary therapies can actually achieve these goals? Are you being truly honest and realistic with your expectations?

There's only one requirement for this exercise: honesty. Whether your expectations match the goals I have listed is irrelevant. It *is* important for you to be completely open and candid with yourself so the answers that form are right for you. It may help to ask a trusted friend to assist you with this exercise. Often, being asked these questions by someone else forces you to be more honest with your answers.

Don't limit yourself to the more "acceptable" or "doable" goals for complementary therapy. While these may bring you a temporary sense of security and may even be fruitful, they won't lead to your full hopes. There is nothing more self-defeating for cancer survivors than feeling that time and energy have been wasted. Allow time for your answers to reveal themselves, even if it means being in that squirmy, squishy, uncomfortable place of unknowing. Clarity will come, and along with it the conviction that you are doing exactly what you need to do.

■ EXERCISE 2: Setting Your Parameters:
An Honest Look at Limitations
Cancer can help you to know yourself better. Living with a life-threatening illness helped me to clarify what I really cherished in life. It motivated me to pursue the goals I wanted to meet while I still could. It both simplified and

complicated my life. In the midst of coping with doctors, treatment decisions, and family and friends, my own wishes became much clearer.

When you're deciding whether to create an integrated treatment plan, it is important to explore what you are willing to do to incorporate complementary medicine into your healing. The following exercise of setting your parameters and priorities makes you more conscious of your limits and helps to further define your relationship with complementary therapies. It also gives you a more realistic idea of how these therapies will—or won't—fit into your life.

For this exercise, put aside for a moment your misgivings about trying complementary medicine and focus on what you honestly feel *you* can do. Ask yourself the following questions:

- How far am I willing to go in my search for complementary medicine?
- How important is it compared with everything else going on? Is it my top priority? What value do I place on conventional versus complementary treatment?
- How much money am I willing to spend on complementary care?
- How much time do I expect to spend researching therapies?
- How much time do I wish to spend taking treatments?
- How far am I willing to travel? Out of my state? Out of the country? Overseas? How often?
- Do I need family support? My physician's concurrence? If I don't receive it, am I willing to continue? To keep my choices or complementary care from them, if necessary? How much stress will that cause? Would I need to change doctors?

- Do I want friends or family to help me research therapies? If so, how much of the information gathering am I willing to let go of? Can I accept their advice?
- Can I put up with the impact of lifestyle changes? How do I feel about minor alterations to my habits, such as taking vitamins and supplements? About major changes, such as traveling one hour each way for a healing treatment, or following a rigid diet? Can I deal with only one kind of change, or both?
- Am I willing to put up with possibly uncomfortable or awkward side effects, like intestinal upset or changes in skin color?

One woman I know found that her priorities changed when she began to research her complementary options. "When I was first diagnosed, I relied heavily on family and friends to research my medical treatment because it was so difficult for me emotionally. I took the information in pieces, as I could handle it. But with complementary therapy, I found I wanted to do it all. I had to cut back on some of the therapies pretty early on because it was exhausting to explore them all at the same time. I found it hard to keep up my complementary therapy schedule while on chemotherapy because I was trying too much at once. But as I researched different treatments, it became pretty clear which ones I wanted to keep and which to cut back."

■ EXERCISE 3: Visualizing Lifestyle Changes

The above are some of the more practical questions you need to ask yourself. But there is a deeper layer you need to sort through as you make your decisions. Try to imagine integrating complementary treatments into your life: the adjustments to your schedule, the impact on family, the financial commitment. How does it make you feel?

Does it feel as if you're burdening everyone and restricting yourself? Or do you feel as if you're taking charge and doing what you can to keep yourself healthy—and therefore it's a small price to pay?

Both answers may present themselves, but try to sit with them and see if one outweighs the other. If complementary therapy feels more like a burden than a blessing, it doesn't necessarily mean that you won't try it—but perhaps you'll do it in more manageable doses.

You might find it useful to compare your answers with the expectations you identified in the first exercise, so your thinking doesn't become more conflicted. For example, after answering these questions, sit awhile with your feelings and reflect on whether they seem to support your primary goal. If you're uncomfortable, adjustments or further examination may be needed in one area or the other, until it "feels right."

■ EXERCISE 4: "What If?"

Try on some worst-case scenarios as well: Imagine going into a healer's office and subjecting yourself to treatments that may dredge up strong emotions, or leave you feeling cheated because you didn't feel a thing. Some treatments initially make you feel worse instead of better. Others progress for a time and then seem to turn back on themselves or stop working altogether. Using complementary therapy takes a lot of faith, even if you have a fair amount of knowledge about the particular therapy you're using.

How much proof will you require of a particular therapy's efficacy before you try it? How much faith do you need in the process? In the healer? In your body and your ability to "read it"? Is there anything you can think of that would make you more comfortable in trying complementary therapy? If so, what would it be?

Now, imagine deciding *not* to try complementary therapy. You're going to stick strictly with your doctor's regimen and just get through it. Or imagine you have fin-
ished therapy and go back to life as you knew it before
cancer. How does that scenario make you feel? Is it
important to you to try complementary therapy? Why?
Can you be at peace with yourself if you don't try it?

REMOVING ROADBLOCKS

I hope that the exercises you have just completed have
given you a clearer sense of your hopes and plans for
complementary therapy. But there can still be a very
unsettling feeling when you think about actually *starting*
treatments. For many, getting through the very real fears
we have of trying anything so unfamiliar can be the most
daunting task of all.

Rumors flourish in the general and medical press
regarding complementary therapy. It's difficult for many
of us to step into the swirling whirlpool of controversy
over these treatments, especially when we feel so vulnerable. Yet we have so much at stake and we feel that whatever may lead us to better health should be considered.
As one survivor of recurrent metastatic breast cancer puts
it, "From my initial diagnosis, I've been a stage IV. I felt
that put me in a different category; I had to pull out all
the stops because I was fighting an uphill battle. For me,
it was more fearful to choose only the conventional
route."

The process of deciding whether to use complementary therapy (and which treatments to use) can paralyze us
into a state of unhealthy fear and indecision. This kind of
"clutching" can be an unnecessary source of stress that
can hamper our efforts to heal. The only way I knew to
free myself was to identify each of my concerns and try
to work through them with objectivity and compassion.

Facing your fears is never easy, but it can be liberating to release them and free up more energy for your healing. Clearly, you are not alone in your fears. We've all had them. So let's walk through these worries together.

ROADBLOCK NO. 1: **Appearing Desperate**
Complementary therapy has been commonly viewed as frivolous, a lark for those "worried well" who have the time and money to dabble in the latest scheme to reverse aging, reduce stress, or improve well-being. While many proponents of complementary therapy are not taken seriously (eyes tend to roll when someone healthy announces he is trying the latest trend), it is a different matter altogether when someone with cancer considers it. Questions abound about whether the person really knows what he is doing. The general assumption is that he is at the end of his rope or that he's searching for cures that may prove useless or worsen his condition. There is mounting evidence, however, that these assumptions are wrong. One recent study reported that their research confirms that "the stereotype that terminally ill, desperate, uneducated patients use CAM [complementary/alternative medicine] is inaccurate."[1] Increasingly, cancer survivors are clarifying their reasons for choosing complementary therapy, becoming realistic about its strengths and limitations (and their own), and doing their homework. When complementary cancer care is explored with caution and purpose (and with a commitment to regularly reevaluate treatment decisions), the likelihood of appearing desperate lessens. Yes, you are taking a risk. But for many of us with relatively unstudied or "difficult" cancers, the risks are not all that different from choosing conventional or experimental medical treatment.

ROADBLOCK NO. 2: Being "In Charge"

While conventional medical care is managed by professionals, *you* are capable of managing a lot more of your complementary care than you might think. That's not just my opinion. It's been repeatedly demonstrated to me through my own experience and that of other cancer survivors. We have successfully combined numerous and varied therapies, often coordinating treatments alongside our medical care—sometimes even combining conventional and complementary treatments—while educating our physicians and healers on how it can be done. Being in charge of your own care can be energizing as you become comfortable with both developing your treatment plan and the treatments themselves.

Of course, there is a learning curve that goes along with selecting and working with complementary therapies for cancer, whether you are already familiar with them or not. And wasting time and money on unsuccessful or unnecessary conventional procedures, incompetent health professionals, and the like seems somehow more acceptable than doing the same with complementary therapies. This sort of convoluted thinking only adds unneeded pressure to "get it right the first time."

Instead, with some work, you can develop a treatment plan regardless of whether you have had experience with complementary therapies. The powerful treatment plans I've seen have been created by people who decided what was most important to them, carefully investigated their options, and pursued complementary therapy with a deep and personal commitment to their healing.

ROADBLOCK NO. 3:
Resistance from Loved Ones and Health Providers

It's only natural that family and friends are concerned about your complementary choices. Everyone wants a positive outcome for you. And most people want to put their trust only in a proven medical course of treatment, no matter how grueling it is.

But they are not you.

They cannot know the isolation you feel, how cut-off you can become from your spirit. They cannot know the overpowering need to do something for yourself when you are feeling so overtaken by the cancer, by medical treatments, by all the uncertainty. For me, no matter how much I believed in my medical treatment and how grateful I was to my doctors, it was still physically torturous and emotionally draining. For fifteen months I felt as if I had shelved my true self to assume the role of patient. I found that complementary therapy could help me feel whole again in a way conventional treatment couldn't match. I felt more integrated when dealing with complementary practitioners who worked with me as myself, not as "cancer patient." I did not fault my doctors for this identification but rather the impersonal nature of the structure in which most medical care is provided. While I felt assured I was receiving the best medical care available, I needed to become more connected to my healing on an intimate, conscious level. For me, the best way to make this connection was through complementary treatment. I had to do this for myself, and I managed to convey this need to my physicians, family, and friends.

It's important to share your conventional medicine experiences with your loved ones, as well. They can be more supportive if they are aware of how you feel about your prognosis, your treatment choices, and your doctors and medical care—much of which they may not know or understand as well as you do. Share with them what you have learned about complementary therapies, both the good and the bad. Dismiss some, select others, and marvel at the various options. Demonstrate that there are choices, and that you aren't just blindly thrashing around in the world of alternative medicine. Discuss with them the knowledge and experience you've gained. With cancer treatment, everyone lives with uncertainty. The trick is learning how to come to terms with it, whether it comes packaged as conventional or complementary.

"I knew I was undergoing a tremendous lifestyle change by using complementary medicine," says a survivor. "But my family hadn't necessarily signed up for it. So it was really good to tell them of my level of commitment—what was happening for me—and hear what that meant for them and for us as a family."

I think it can be even more frightening for some of us to deal with our physicians, who may be averse to the use of complementary therapy. Many cancer patients express an interest in getting information on complementary therapies from their physicians, but just as many feel they can't discuss the topic with them. Many cancer survivors' stories of using complementary therapies are peppered with discouraging reports of doctors who were angry with or dismissive of their patient's use of such treatments. For every doctor who demonstrates interest or support for complementary cancer therapies, there seem to be several who question, discourage, forbid, or mock them. It can be very stressful to feel you aren't being heard or taken seriously. So numerous are these accounts that cancer patients using complementary therapies sometimes feel they must abide by a "don't ask/don't tell" policy. A recent study of breast cancer patients using complementary therapy showed that only 54 percent discussed their complementary choices with their physicians.[7] Poor communication is a common reason cited by patients for switching to another physician.

While many patients won't broach the topic of complementary therapy with their physicians for fear of alienating them, some gingerly test the waters. Whatever the response, if it's not what they had hoped for, it may be enough to discourage them from trying complementary care, or from sharing their choices with their physicians in the future.

On the bright side, times are changing and physicians are becoming more open to integrative medicine. Medical oncologist Carolyn Hendricks, M.D., observes, "Physicians are more willing to combine the best of clinical and complementary therapy in treating patients with cancer. Complementary cancer treatments are already taking a greater role in palliative care. While it's still patient-driven, physicians *are* coming around. It's a *fact*." At the least, cancer patients' use of complementary therapies is challenging oncologists to improve their relationships with their patients. In a recent editorial addressed primarily to fellow oncologists, Harold J. Burstein, M.D., Ph.D., of the Dana Farber Cancer Institute, acknowledged the prevalence and application of complementary cancer care. He pointed out the opportunity oncologists have to communicate better with their patients and to be more attentive to their needs, sharing in the cancer experience on a deeper, more meaningful level.[8]

I was fortunate to find physicians who welcomed my attitude toward integrative medicine. While not experienced in complementary therapies, they were curious, encouraging, and open to information on the treatments I was using or considering. Certainly the *ideal* of having physicians who are knowledgeable in several complementary modalities and aggressively investigating others for me did not eventuate. But I was never laughed at, dismissed, or frightened into abandoning my choices. Rather, our relationship of mutual respect and trust assured that we would find the right answers together. I believe it made all the difference in my response to conventional treatments.

That difference was based on *open communication,* which gave me a clear understanding of how I would be supported. You need to know where people stand with you, whether they are doctors, other health practitioners, your family, or friends. It's important to see who's standing by you and who may be discouraging you, and determine whether that perception is real or imagined.

One woman, when asking her doctor about the relationship of exercise and nutrition to cancer, was dismissed with, "I don't know anything about that, but it's irrelevant." She decided that her doctor didn't need to be her only resource for medical information. Ultimately she changed doctors because she felt this one wasn't a good match and did not operate at the level of involvement she wanted from her caregiver.

Another cancer patient was recovering from surgery when her doctor stopped by. She told him of her desire to strengthen her immune system using complementary therapy. He responded that she "might as well use astrology" for all the good it would do her. While at first she was disappointed and frustrated with his attitude, she was ultimately grateful. "It forced me to articulate my commitment to complementary therapy and my desire to participate more fully in my healing. It showed me that I would not give anyone else sole responsibility for my getting better, and that I could appreciate his skills and strengths while bringing my talents and resources to my healing as well. Our disagreement and different approaches ultimately strengthened our relationship."

If you find that resistance doesn't lessen over time or with open communication, you need to take into account how much this opposition will affect your desire to pursue complementary treatment. Your choice may put you at odds with your family, friends, or health care team throughout your treatment or as you recover. If so, you may have to make a decision about whether to continue with your complementary care or perhaps find another physician who will support your position. It might be useful to tell your "opposition" how their behavior affects you; knowing that may help lessen their resistance. Or perhaps you can reach a compromise with them, such as agreeing to a discussion about your choices when they feel your safety is at risk or on some sort of regular basis, as a way of "checking in."

I don't recommend hiding your use of complementary therapy; I believe this only generates more stress for you. I have seen others engage in closeted complementary treatments, believing it was their only choice. Ultimately, the option is yours. But before you start, ask yourself if hiding your treatments is really the best—or only—way for you. Your motivation for using complementary therapy is to help heal yourself, so it is important to make your decision from faith and not fear, even in the face of resistance.

ROADBLOCK NO. 4: Expense

This particular roadblock has stopped many from exploring complementary therapies; unfortunately, these treatments can be costly. While some of these therapies are now covered (at least partially) by insurance, sadly, most of them are not.

It is also becoming more common to find physicians practicing complementary medicine who participate in managed care plans. Usually, however, they are practicing at physicians' prices. Even after insurance reimbursement, the cost can be comparable to out-of-pocket payments to holistic practitioners.

The issue of cost can dampen your enthusiasm for complementary therapy or even become the determining factor in some treatment decisions. Several survivors I spoke with admitted that money spent on complementary therapy is an ongoing concern. One man observed that he had spent thousands of dollars on treatments not covered by his insurance, "but they offered me hope for a possible remission, and I knew I had to do whatever I could to achieve that goal. It was different, though, spending more money on complementary therapies that did not seem as essential. I knew I would have to choose carefully." Another survivor acknowledged that "for me it was going to be 'whatever it takes.' Trial and error was an important part of the process, and I knew there would be some waste, both in terms of time and money. I decided that would be okay. But I'm still waiting for the dust to settle financially—if it ever does."

Pricing practices among complementary therapists have some common traits with those among conventional health providers. But there are significant differences as well. For instance, I found that, for the most part, practitioners in my immediate area offered competitive prices for their professional services. Like physicians, their fees seemed a fair reflection of their skill, training, and the quality of the treatment provided. Many seemed to actively *under*value their services, however, especially when compared with the very generous amount of time they offered, sometimes twice as long as scheduled. It was also not uncommon for practitioners to offer me an introduction to treatment at no cost, which is certainly a change from traditional health care practices.

Complementary products can be, in some cases, more costly than services, which certainly forced me to prioritize. But again, some distributors of these products were often very generous, and would discount products if I committed to a certain length of time or bought in bulk. Keep in mind that you will be spending a significant amount of time finding the best complementary therapies for you.

Giving products and services trial periods before committing to them is often a wise course. It can help to reduce the anxiety of feeling that you are pouring significant amounts of money into something you're not sure will work.

A creative approach to financing complementary care may help you to reduce your concerns about cost. I was fortunate enough to work with practitioners who were very sensitive to the stresses and constraints of being a cancer patient. When I tried out a therapy and felt strongly that it was beneficial but found the cost prohibitive, I would muster up the courage to have an honest discussion about it. I found many of my healers to be very empathetic and generous in their willingness to explore creative financing with me. We might slow down, for instance, the schedule of treatments to reduce monthly payments. Sliding scales were negotiable. Sometimes, reduced fees for a fixed length of time, or in exchange for a commitment to long-term treatment, would be offered. Some practitioners are open to bartering, whereby they agree to trade services. And training programs for practitioners often welcome clients at a reduced fee for their students to practice on. For example, I found substantially reduced prices with several massage schools and individual apprentice energy workers.

While I'd like to lessen your fears about the cost of complementary care, I don't want to paint a picture of a free ride. Rather, the vast majority of practitioners I personally dealt with and interviewed for this book were sympathetic. They acknowledged the difference between clients with less serious chronic conditions and cancer patients accessing multiple services and products, at a time when medical costs may be mounting. Many were open to flexibility and creativity in how they were compensated.

In being creative, you may wish to explore other, less costly sources for complementary care. Look for programs on complementary medicine at your local hospital. More are beginning to offer classes on various therapies for a nominal fee. They can be a good introduction to a modality, and perhaps a way to meet local practitioners and other survivors interested in complementary care. Health fairs and conferences on complementary treatments frequently give demonstrations or offer services on-site. And you can benefit from several complementary practices with little to no financial investment. Many survivors form their own informal support, spirituality, or writing groups (as well as research groups to exchange information on complementary treatments) and exercise or meditation groups. For instance, one support group I joined was initiated by two breast cancer survivors who were introduced to each other by their physician. Unable to find a support group on their own, they took each other out to lunch and launched "The Lunch Bunch." Within a few years, "The Bunch" became a haven to over fifty survivors, who meet each week over lunch for camaraderie and to discuss topics of interest raised by invited speakers.

You may at some point, wish to "launch out" on your own. Other survivors I know have received professional instruction on guided imagery and visualization, meditative practices such as qi gong or tai chi, or exercise programs such as yoga, but once they gained confidence, they instituted their own practice, purchasing tapes or designing programs they could follow by themselves.

ROADBLOCK NO. 5:
Scientific Efficacy/Health Concerns
The fear that complementary therapy will do more harm than good may be a very real one, especially when your health is already compromised as a result of cancer. As one complementary therapy user acknowledged, "You're

used to dealing with disease from a scientific perspective, so dealing with the unknowns of complementary therapy is scary." As I mentioned earlier, many of the claims made by complementary therapy proponents are scientifically unproven and most success stories are anecdotal. The field of complementary medicine is making progress in conducting reproducible research, but it is still evolving.

It is important to keep in mind that complementary and alternative medicine indicators of success are often experiential and sensory, and can be difficult to measure. Medical treatment is generally more targeted—procedures and drugs are designed for specific diseases or conditions—and so is better served by scientific evaluation.

As one practitioner puts it, "With allopathic medicine, 'feel good' isn't good enough; with complementary medicine, 'feel good' is all there is. The two speak different languages and are different cultures, so seeking integrative care is essentially a cross-cultural experience."

Many complementary modalities have clearly enjoyed thousands of years of use by millions around the world, and public acceptance of these modalities is growing in the United States. However, the lack of scientific evidence supporting complementary therapies is still a barrier for both practitioners and patients, and can make the decision to use these treatments more labor-intensive. This is particularly true for those who are research-oriented.

I found two ways to work through this fear. First, I gained a deeper appreciation for the complexity of cancer and its unique expression in each individual. I know that for many of us, statistics can be a real source of comfort and a reason for hope during particularly difficult times of treatment. For me they were not. The statistics for my type of cancer condemned me to die within eighteen months of diagnosis. Even if I beat those daunting odds, I discovered that I still had only a 40 percent chance to survive for five years. In months of telephone searches and advertisement inquiries in support of my medical treatment decisions, I found largely anecdotal reports. There was little solid ground, nor was there much solace or optimism in my research. As a result I concluded that, in many ways, my decisions regarding conventional cancer treatment had to be just as intuitive as my choices of complementary therapies.

Second, I wasn't reconciled to closing my eyes and picking the complementary therapy *du jour* as a way of easing my fear. I felt I owed it to myself to be as meticulous in selecting my complementary therapy as I had been in selecting my conventional treatment, despite the lack of information. I used the "stop, look, and listen" approach in assuaging my fears. Before I started any treatment, I took the time to get comfortable with the modality. I conducted research to find out how much was or wasn't known. I sought out other cancer survivors and listened to them relate their personal experience with the treatment. I questioned practitioners who could best tell me the pros and cons of the treatment, including its compatibility with conventional therapy and asked for documentation of treatment safety and efficacy. And I looked for the "holes." How reliable were the sources? What was said and—just as importantly—what was left unsaid?

Whether you find reason to believe a particular therapy's claims or not, the final step is going inward and finding out why you are trying a particular treatment. You may find you are comfortable with simply doing a cursory search, talking to a few survivors and providers, or casually asking around, rather than conducting in-depth research. Or you may just rely on intuition. The soul-searching you do regarding your intentions and limitations will also help. Only you know what it takes to achieve your level of comfort.

"I knew there wasn't enough research information about how effective these [complementary] therapies were to make me feel 100 percent comfortable, but that didn't mean they wouldn't work or ultimately be the best option for me," said one survivor. "I thought whatever the cure really is for cancer, it too is still in the 'unproven' category right now."

Taking some time to investigate your conventional treatment options can also be important. (Of course, you will need to consider the urgency of your particular situation.) Current cancer treatments sometimes carry with them severe side effects that can be life-changing. We are led to believe that conventional medicine offers the best chance for survival, but as one physician-acupuncturist and cancer survivor notes, "That belief needs to be challenged, or at least not taken for granted, because statistics don't always back it up."

In other words, scrutinize *any* treatment offered, whether complementary or conventional, and if you feel you need a little more time, ask for it. Don't be afraid to ask for second—and even third—opinions. Follow your intuition as well as your intellect. Keep your eye on the goal of healing yourself and don't shortchange the process you need to go through in order to make your decision. Consider risk, but don't be intimidated by it. You have more power than you think!

ROADBLOCK NO. 6:

Traveling Away from Home (Separation from Loved Ones)

In your search for complementary therapies you may find several that appeal to you but are only available outside your area of residence. While location may seem irrelevant, the exotic nature of these therapies can cause even more apprehension when they have to be administered in an unfamiliar place. Travel costs, combined with the cost of the treatment itself, can make this dilemma even more stressful.

One way to overcome this roadblock is to do your research on the treatment, practitioner, and facility. Know ahead of time any contraindications, side effects, complications, and risks to health, and discuss these with your physician. You must have faith that this treatment will help you in some way; this is a bigger step than a local intervention. Ask for references and talk to those cancer survivors who have traveled there for treatment. If possible, take an orientation trip. See if the therapy can be administered closer to home, either in whole or in part by a trained practitioner or physician. Sometimes you or a caregiver can be taught the procedure, thereby reducing your time away.

If you must be away from home for an extended period, try to arrange for someone to go with you as morale booster and advocate. One cancer patient who traveled out of the country for treatment put it well: "Extreme situations call for extreme measures. Going with my spouse kept hope alive for me."

Break down the time spent away from home into manageable pieces if you can, scheduling a convenient time for the treatment to minimize disruption to you and your family. And always leave yourself an escape clause, even if it's a pseudo-one. "I did have the notion that if I got there and didn't like what I saw, I would leave," said one survivor. "All I would be out was money and we're talking about my life! So each day would have to pass the smell test and make sense or I would be outta' there."

ROADBLOCK NO. 7: Making the Wrong Choice

This particular fear is one that's near and dear to my heart. For instance, I avoid large stores because there are far too many choices for my comfort level. On one hand,

I was so eager to try complementary medicine that I wanted to do everything, all at once. But I also worried about making the wrong choice. It was a real struggle for me to avoid being frozen by my inability to decide what was best, or trapped into pursuing every possibility for healing.

I found myself comparing my choices with those of other survivors, which did me no good at all. I was stunned by what I would call the alternative "marathoners": those people who were relentless in their pursuit of complementary therapies. They were walking encyclopedias on fifty different treatments, savvy in reaching researchers from all over the country, always familiar with whatever you were contemplating. They had "been there, done that." I envied their seasoned attitude and their confidence in dismissing a therapy as unsuitable. And I was particularly anxious to know their secret formula: exactly what combination of therapies did they pursue? In what sequence did they try them, and for how long, to achieve such great results? What were they trying now? Was this option better than the one that was recommended to me the week before? Where could I get it? I felt I was in a race in which I had started late and would never catch up.

Now, I really *did* feel desperate. While I knew I was gaining by the experience of these survivors, I sabotaged myself with self-doubt in response to their confidence. I had to learn to stop competing with them and instead receive whatever wisdom I could, trusting that it was what I needed at the moment.

While you may feel like a novice diving into a sea of seasoned triathlon swimmers, the best advice I can give you is to go ahead and take the plunge. Those already using complementary therapies for cancer are a tremendous resource of information and experience and will teach you a great deal—not only about therapies, but about love, courage, creativity, and perseverance. And also about how there are no "wrong choices." The support of those who have been there before you is one of the greatest gifts you can receive from this illness. I think of my own initial support group: Maxine, Gunnell, Bernice, Jean, and Maria. Through their wisdom, humor, and strength of spirit, they gave me the push I needed to search for my own answers. In their love and grace I was held and my heaviness of spirit was lifted. I will be forever grateful to them, and consider them to be my healers as much as any practitioner I used for treatment.

You will find your own angels, as I did mine. If from your deepest place you state your intent to help yourself heal and ask for help in finding your way, that help will come in truly amazing ways. As one cancer survivor put it, "I had to learn to trust my intuition as a suitable decision-making path. When things are trying to get your attention, they'll let you know. You just need to trust that what you need to do will find *you*."

ROADBLOCK NO. 8: Not Doing Enough

Many of us struggle with the fear of not doing enough on a daily basis. It's a natural reaction to feeling overwhelmed, and yet it runs deeper than that, fueling the compulsive drive to try everything. When this takes over, developing a healing plan can change from a creative process of self-discovery into a tortuous search that never ends. I've coached many survivors who have a strong desire to help themselves heal, but are held back by their guilt. They feel entirely responsible for their progress. They think *they* are in charge of whether they go into remission or relapse, and are, therefore, obligated to try everything as soon as possible. I, too, lived in that space for a while—before it drove me absolutely crazy. I have never been one to make instant decisions, and after trying this mindset on for size, I found myself asking, "How can anyone possibly heal under this much pressure?" Over time I found that I wouldn't die if I didn't start a particular therapy immediately, or ever at all. And it was okay to let go of some complementary therapies that just didn't seem right for me.

I absolved myself from feeling responsible for any relapse that might occur. There's a healthy sense of taking charge, and then there's an out-of-control desire to be in control, and I was in the latter category. A little self-forgiveness and compassion were in order! Nurturing yourself is critical to healing. Give yourself room to be human; acknowledge that this is all new, that seeming "mistakes" and "dead ends" can lead you to a truth you might not have discovered otherwise.

Your real challenge is not simply to pick the best treatments for you, but to keep your eyes, ears, and heart open. Observe yourself as you listen to other survivors, do your research, and begin to get answers. Record not only what you hear and where you heard it, but your feelings about it. Go back and redo the exercises on expectations and parameters to help you figure out where you stand each time you ponder a potential treatment.

It's not as daunting as it first appears. Over time you'll know what you need before you take action. At some point you'll be able to see how it all falls into place: every decision, every doubt, every "failure"...and how they lead you to the next success. You can learn from it all. And it's wonderful when you can appreciate the beauty of the process itself.

It helps to remember that progress isn't always linear, so you may find yourself taking three steps forward and two back. It is very easy to get lost in the details and be overcome by the sheer volume of information and the endless combinations of therapies successfully used by others. Most people become overwhelmed at some point. Slow down and try to keep your focus on the goal of building your very *own* healing plan. You really do have all the time you need—on a much deeper level than most of us ever understand. When the process feels out of control, try to trust that you have the answers inside, even if it feels as if you need to organize an archeological dig through your subconscious to reach them.

And *please*: ask for help. This is one hurdle that seems to be really tough for cancer survivors. None of us has even half of all the answers. We are so used to the illusion of being "competent, independent adults," in control of our destinies. Then cancer shows us what an illusion it has been. Even after our rude awakening, we continue to insist on going it alone. But help is all around us; it's there for the asking. As one survivor observed, "All you have to do is take one step on this path and the universe rolls out to greet you."

Send your intention out into the world, and ask for help—both out loud, to those who will hear you, and in prayer. I guarantee that the response you get will amaze, frustrate, delight, and confuse you!

And in precisely the ways you need, it can heal you.

CHAPTER 4

CREATING YOUR PLAN

Now that you've faced your concerns about using complementary therapy, you're ready to roll up your sleeves and start developing and implementing your treatment plan. This has been the most difficult chapter to write in the entire book, because I know it presents you with the most challenging part of building your plan: selecting treatments and choosing practitioners. But before you go running for the door, I want to tell you something that I hope will help you to relax. This chapter will simply reinforce what you already know at some level; you won't find major revelations here, but instead a guide to making choices and building a well-grounded plan. Hopefully, you'll be reminded of some practical truths—the kind that are so easy to forget in the midst of personal chaos—that will steer you clear of some of the more common pitfalls.

What's your investigational style? How can you organize your time and find good sources of information to help you select the right modalities? What decision-making process will best allow you to choose your practitioners wisely? We'll explore each one. Along the way, I've highlighted some "shopping tips" that may seem simplistic at first glance, but are critical to remember throughout the process in order to make your life easier.

Now, on to the matter at hand...

WHAT'S YOUR SHOPPING STYLE?
Shopping: people seem either to love it or to hate it. I've

never been much of a shopper. Oh, I enjoy it once in a while, but I prefer the streamlined approach: I only go when I absolutely have to. I preselect my store, slip in, make my purchase, and exit, mission accomplished. I marvel at people who love to spend a day cruising the malls. They actually see it as a form of recreation, and return from shopping energized, even triumphant! If I spend more than two hours shopping, I need a nap.

Shopping for complementary therapies is no different. There appear to be two camps: the adrenaline-pumped explorers, ready to set forth into the unknown, feeling exhilarated, excited, confident, empowered. Then there are those who view it all as tedious, murky, and basically a lot of hard work. They'd rather leave the job to the "professional shoppers."

While there is no particular advantage in one style over the other, it helps to have a good sense of your preferred shopping style and what makes you comfortable when looking for complementary cancer care. When dealing with a life-threatening illness, you may find that you want to combine both styles. There is a common tendency to exhaust yourself doing all sorts of investigating, sifting, and sorting of information when searching for complementary treatments. Even if you enjoy shopping, you can feel overwhelmed in these circumstances. It can be frustrating to find yourself compelled to do extensive research when you are the type who hates to shop. Or to find that you've done all the investigative work, but still must rely on intuition, an approach you're not entirely comfortable with.

You can end up making the decision-making process more difficult than it has to be by trying to fit yourself into a particular mold. Keep in mind that there are many different ways to select treatments and practitioners. Just try to go with your natural flow. If you shop primarily by instinct, great. If you need to do some research first, then have a good idea of how much information you need to make a decision. If you can delegate some of the research, even better; it can be a tremendous amount of work. Just don't let the subject matter force you into an investigative method that you're not comfortable with. And know that you don't need to "shop 'til you drop." That's not what this process is all about. I'm writing this book in the hope that it will save you some precious time and energy that is better spent toward the goal of healing yourself. So make this material work for *you*.

GETTING ORGANIZED

If you have a sense that it's a very big ocean out there, you're right. You can spend a lot of time and effort trying to cover it all, or you can set your sights on what seems a priority for you.

I found it helpful to impose some structure on my shopping for treatments. This allowed me to break it down from one enormous mass of therapies into identifiable areas that would be in alignment with my goal of supporting myself through treatment and enhancing my recovery. My apathy in exploring complementary therapies was partly due to my inability to focus—compliments of chemotherapy—which added to my natural aversion to shopping. By making general categories of complementary modalities that I thought would be useful, I began to grasp what I needed to do and felt more confident that out of this mass I could shape a personal treatment plan.

SHOPPING TIP NO. 1:
Focus Your Efforts on Areas That Will Best Support You
Determine which areas you think will best support you in your healing. Focusing on these will break down your

research into manageable pieces. It's like planning a vacation. You start with what you feel you want: rest and relaxation, learning something new, or challenging yourself physically. Then you focus on where you want to go. Beach or mountains? Warm or cold? Urban or rural? With others or alone? You begin to shape your efforts according to what you and your body want in order to get to a better place than where you are now.

Others have done admirable jobs of categorizing complementary therapies into clusters. While these may be helpful to many, when I read them I still didn't have a clue what some of them might mean to me! I only had a vague idea of what I felt I needed, but from that I was able to identify five areas that I designated as my support systems for healing. These areas seem to be a useful starting point for many. You may find they work for you, or serve as an inspiration to help you design a different system altogether.

Healing Support Systems

- **NUTRITION:** Included here is anything ingested that would enhance my immune system or physically strengthen my body. As I proceeded, I found that "nutrition" involved significant changes in diet as well as adding nutritional supplements, herbs, and teas.
- **EXERCISE:** I tried to find better ways to incorporate activity into my daily routine, acknowledging the physical and emotional benefits of exercise and its effect on my immune system. I went beyond the concept of exercise as a dreaded MDR (minimum daily requirement) to fight off total lethargy. I found I enjoyed becoming creative with movement, choosing from a variety of new activities that helped me to step out of my cancer and appreciate how powerful exercise could be in my healing.

- **EMOTIONAL SUPPORT/STRESS REDUCTION:** I defined this support as any activity that would facilitate better access to my true self and the release of intense and stressful emotions. I used visualization, guided imagery, affirmations, and meditation; participated in support groups and individual therapy; and made a commitment to saying what I meant and meaning what I said on a more regular basis. And I began a deeper exploration of joy: what it meant, where it was, and how to have more of it in my life.
- **ENERGY WORK:** I set about finding and maintaining balance through structural (body) work and energy healing. Some of my treatments included polarity therapy, shiatsu massage, Rolfing, yoga, and other techniques I felt would align and strengthen my life force energy.
- **SPIRITUAL GUIDANCE:** I became more conscious of a strong desire to nourish my soul, deepen my relationship to God, and stay connected to the earth in this extremely challenging time. I found a healer whom I believed would guide me toward the spiritual growth I longed for.

What's important here is for you to decide which supports you need, since everyone has a slightly different approach. For instance, one breast cancer survivor explained how she organized herself: "When I first began looking at complementary therapies, I had no idea what I was doing. I just put one little paw ahead of the other little paw. I had to deal with the resources where I lived, and so began to create a template for myself, based on five categories: diet, nutrition, and exercise; mind/body issues; natural herbal remedies; pharmacological treatments; and lifestyle changes. Then, within each of these categories, I looked for the obvious 'no-brainers' that I could begin to incorporate into my plan. For example, with my diet, I chose to stop consuming meat and dairy products. That's how I got started."

I found I instantly connected to the five categories I had identified. When I began looking into various treatments, I found that while there was plenty of overlap in assigning therapies to my categories, I could at least make an initial cut based on whether they fit into my healing support systems. In other words, it was a good place to start and gave me a feeling of order. I noticed I received more helpful responses when I asked about a particular category (like nutrition or energy work) than when I asked for general help. And focusing on these categories helped to keep my little mental gremlins at bay.

GAIN YOUR DEGREE
WHILE BATTLING CANCER!

One thing about complementary therapy: looking into all the modalities can sure take your mind off your cancer for a while. There is so much to learn that it can feel like your first year in a doctoral program. Actually, some cancer survivors, myself included, have found new vocations in exploring healing alternatives.

Most of us get started by just diving in, gathering information wherever found. But you have to find your balance between information overload and the amount and kind of data *you* need to reach an informed decision and take action. Don't hesitate to call upon trusted friends to help you exhaust the possibilities, instead of exhausting yourself. While many survivors aren't comfortable handing over the research to someone else, others find it invaluable. "The most important thing to me was having someone else do the research and feed the information to me as I needed it, because I couldn't possibly digest everything out there all at once," reported a seasoned user of complementary treatments.

A rich variety of resources abounds for gathering information for your treatment plan. The Appendix and Modality sections contain selected resources that offer valuable assistance to those searching for complementary cancer care. Each kind of resource has its unique strengths and drawbacks, so it's important to know how to use each one.

Books and Tapes

There are an abundance of wonderful general guides to complementary and alternative medicine. It might be useful to acquire some for personal reference, to turn to as needed. Often these books list sources for more specific information on each treatment described that may lead you to practitioners as well. The Modalities section and the Appendix also contain recommendations for books on specific complementary therapies or complementary cancer care, which often describe every conceivable treatment, and then some.

An abundance of alternative medicine journals and newsletters will provide you with the latest on popular and promising therapies, although their primary focus may not be cancer. It is a real challenge to keep abreast of new therapies and approaches to complementary cancer treatment, particularly through published material. It's a dynamic field and more is being discovered, changed, or refuted every day. I would love to see a "What's Hot/What's Not" list of complementary cancer therapies, but it's not likely. So it's a good idea to check in from time to time. It might help to enlist any bibliophiles you know to be your "research assistants." I consider myself lucky that I have yet to be arrested for loitering in libraries or bookstores!

Audio- and videotapes can give you good insight into—and even hands-on experience with—some treatments. They are a relatively inexpensive way to try tai chi, meditation, yoga, and guided imagery, for instance, or to hear from practitioners or researchers about their modalities. One way to find these tapes is to attend complementary health fairs and conferences. Sometimes the organizers of these events will sell recordings of the proceedings that cover popular therapies or controversial topics, which often include questions from the audience.

Some general contact sources for ordering tapes are listed in the Appendix.

Internet

The Internet is an amazing world offering instant access to complementary care information for the cancer patient, such as introductions to integrative centers, particular healers and modalities, medical databases, research and reports on treatments, and personal stories, to name a few. The availability and variety of information is awe-inspiring in its abundance and frightening in its lack of guidance. Jacqueline Wootton, M.Ed., president and director of the Alternative Medicine Foundation, a nonprofit organization providing balanced, reliable information on alternatives to conventional medicine to researchers and consumers, notes the challenges and rewards for cancer survivors using the Internet in their research.

"The largest single category of inquiries we receive are about cancer. There's an enormous concentration of high-quality information out there on the Internet, but you have to know where to look. In sorting through the web, cancer survivors have a mammoth task in front of them. If people go on-line themselves, they are subject to a lot of commercial information. You need to become editors yourselves, to be able to sift and sort through information, says Wootton.

A common complaint from survivors is the sheer volume of information. The organization of information is also a problem: it can be difficult to come up with a search term that automatically gives you what you need. To illustrate, while writing this chapter, I queried the AltaVista search engine on several complementary cancer terms, and found the number of web pages ranged from 952 to 13,415. Internet searches can be incredibly time-consuming. Many survivors (myself included) find spending hours at the computer screen exhausting rather than exhilarating. But the Internet can provide an amazing array of resources if you're comfortable with it.

Moreover, issues surrounding the quality and reliability of electronic information are not to be taken lightly. Only recently I heard about the first industry-wide ethical and privacy standards for online health sites. As of this writing, research is "only just starting" on developing similar standards for alternative medicine web sites, according to Janlori Goldman of the Health Privacy Project at Georgetown University. It's common these days to see articles in the general press warning Internet users to be wary of what they find, especially in the realm of health care, because information can deceive or confuse readers.

Among the many watchdog organizations for accurate information on the Internet, one of the best is the Health On the Net Foundation (HON) (www.hon.ch). This not-for-profit international Swiss organization was created in 1995. Their mission "is to guide lay persons or non-medical users and medical practitioners to useful and reliable online medical and health information." The foundation also provides international leadership in setting ethical standards for web site developers. Web sites must apply for the priviledge of bearing the HON Code of Conduct (HONcode©) and must pass rigorous scrutiny to be awarded the code. The HONcode is a sort of "stamp of approval" that indicates that the site in question is providing authoritative, trustworthy web-based medical information.

Health information on the Internet is often difficult to access and unreliable, and requires a high reading level to understand. Ms. Wootton advises cancer survivors, in general, to "scrutinize any web site that ends in '.com,' because these sites are focused on selling, and are less likely to be offering clear, impartial information. Educational sites, foundations, and even government sites are good sources for information and research resources. Chat rooms can be useful for getting a balanced view of the pros and cons of treatments, but it's important to remember that these are people swapping stories and are not necessarily experts." As cancer patients, we are particularly vulnerable to misinformation. We can turn that vulnerability into an asset by being particularly thorough in our evaluation of Internet information. (Note: The suggestions presented in Shopping Tip No. 2 can be applied to Internet sources to assess the quality of the information.)

One popular use of the Internet by cancer patients is to connect with other survivors via mailing lists and chat rooms. There are a variety of mailing lists devoted to discussions of specific subjects of interest to cancer patients. These can be accessed using e-mail. Chat rooms offer the opportunity to correspond "live" on-line with other patients and survivors on whatever topic is of interest to the participants. Many cancer web sites will direct you to appropriate chat rooms and listserves.

The Internet has great potential in providing relevant, reliable information on complementary cancer care efficiently, and much is already being offered that will affect how patients make decisions on their health care. But the field is still evolving. While you can be richly rewarded using the Internet to address health concerns, you need to do so with some skepticism and lots of stamina. An avid Internet user advises fellow survivors: "The Internet is a marvelous resource; the caveat is not so much in the vehicle itself, but in the information presented. The ability to discriminate and find your own way is going to be *your* job, which can be good or bad. It's all in how you use it."

Many survivors swear by the Internet; others swear at it. You need to decide whether you want to go down this road at all. If you do, I hope you proceed with a healthy amount of caution and with sharpened critical skills. The Appendix and Modalities sections contain selected web sites to help you get started.

Information Services

Fee-based information services provide cancer patients with the latest information on complementary and conventional therapy options appropriate for their kind of cancer. Information is gathered from a variety of sources, including extensive literature and Internet searches and conferences with alternative and traditional medical experts. Some services, in exchange for pertinent information on your medical condition, will provide you with personalized information that addresses your specific needs. (Some of these services are listed in the Appendix.)

Networking

Exploring complementary cancer therapies can feel like a treasure hunt; there are unexpected gifts to be found by expanding your knowledge through those whom you already trust or will come to rely on. The array of potential therapies and healers is vast, but the community of knowledgeable available people can make the search much more manageable. I found it very reassuring to get recommendations and feedback from people who had personal experience with various modalities of interest. One trusted source—whether a fellow survivor, health provider, caregiver, complementary practitioner, family member, or friend—can make all the difference in pursuing the best treatments for you. One survivor, savvy in networking, said, "When I first began my search, I spoke with a friend who turned me onto *her* friend who was well versed in complementary care. I was thrilled to have that one contact. You only need one name to open the world of alternative therapies to you. That opening may feel the size of a keyhole instead of a barn door, but that opening is all you need."

I consider networking to be a universal skill: if you already know how to find a good repair person through friends, then you're more than halfway there. If you're uncomfortable with or unable to do networking, find a friend who can. Begin with those whom you know and see where they lead you. If they are unable to help you, ask for the name of another person or place that might be able to.

Be as specific as you can with your questions in order to avoid confusion and get solid leads. Look for people and places that have already done some of the legwork for you. You may be able to locate and work with local resource referral groups, alternative health organizations, integrative medical centers, cancer organizations, community alternative publications or local support groups that keep lists of recommended treatments (and perhaps local practitioners). Health fairs, conferences, and lectures on alternative practices (sometimes given at community hospitals) can also be good places to start.

Part of your networking can even include advertising; for instance, I let my doctors know I was interested in meeting other cancer patients who had some experience in complementary care and asked them to pass my name along. I found a cancer newsletter that allowed readers to post queries. Mine brought dozens of responses. Many other survivors network through chat rooms and list services on-line.

You can also try calling complementary practitioners to speak in general about their modality and how it applies to cancer. Hopefully you will end up with good advice, a recommendation for another practitioner, or find yourself talking with someone you want to work with. (See Shopping Tip No. 4 for suggestions on interviewing practitioners.)

Although you will sometimes hit dead-ends in your networking, connecting with the experience and wisdom of others can be transforming in itself, something that far outweighs any difficulties you might encounter. "I've always been nervous about networking," says another survivor. "But getting really good referrals from people I could trust helped enormously. The number of people I draw upon for referrals continues to widen: I constantly try to expand my own network and stay open to others' knowledge."

DON'T FORGET TO KICK THE TIRES

Even though you may have gathered information with wild abandon, the time comes for cautious evaluation. Because most information supporting complementary therapies is still largely anecdotal, you'll need to keep an objective eye and ear as you sift through it all. As has been said, people give more attention to buying a car than to selecting their medical care. May this *not* be true for you. For cancer patients, it's especially important to be discriminating.

SHOPPING TIP NO. 2:

Be Savvy in Your Search and Discriminating in Your Selection

Here are some points to keep in mind when collecting information—regardless of the source—that will hopefully give you a more balanced, accurate picture of the treatments you are considering:

- Look at *who* wrote the information. What are their credentials? Are they reputable? Whom do they represent? What is the quality of the references cited?

- Look at *what* it says. Search for information from scientific literature, preferably peer-reviewed, that supports the use of the treatment of interest. Look for balanced information supported by sound reasoning. Try to find additional studies that support or criticize the treatment that will give you a more realistic picture of the therapy. No single study can claim a cure, whether it is conventional or complementary. Also, finding additional studies of a treatment that support the original findings can strengthen the case for its reliability.

- Look at *how* it's written. Note whether the information appears to be presented in a balanced fashion. Many articles and audiotapes come off as advertisements for treatments. Glowing testimonials from users are given, sometimes with denouncements of conventional treatments or the medical system. Mysterious secret formulas are also sometimes mentioned, or practices are endorsed that cannot be explained to your satisfaction. Trust your instincts: if it doesn't ring true or feels uncomfortable, then put it away.

- Look at *how* others respond to it. Ask around for opinions on the research or information that you've gathered. Has anyone ever heard of it? How popular is it? Physicians, complementary practitioners, and survivors make excellent critics.

- Look at *when* it was written. Information changes constantly with regard to the latest promising therapy for cancer. It's challenging to stay current, but new evidence can be powerful enough sometimes to change a treatment decision. Pay attention to when your information was published, and be on the lookout for addenda to your original sources through the press, the Internet, and your network of professionals and survivors.

■ Look at *why* it was written. Who sponsored the research? Investigate any organizations involved in the study. Is there a hidden agenda or conflict of interest? Do the author(s) or sponsors stand to profit from the promotion of the information?

Be discriminating in your networking as well. Evaluate those who are giving you advice. If they are not trusted friends or recognized experts, look closely. Is their advice based on first-hand experience? Are they being objective? Ask pointed questions to ascertain the depth of their knowledge and breadth of experience. When they are at the choosing stage, many survivors find it useful to ask a trusted friend or health professional to help evaluate their options. Sometimes just having one more person's objective view can be instrumental in making the decision.

Stay in the present with your plan. As I've said earlier, the desire to read all the research and keep up with all the new developments is strong. But the stress of trying to "cover it all" can only impede your healing and perhaps keep you from actually using any complementary therapy. All you can do is educate yourself as best you can and move forward, knowing that you are making an informed decision from what you have been able to learn. You may wish to keep notes in your journal on modalities that you are interested in but not quite comfortable with as yet, remembering that your treatment plan is dynamic. The treatment you reject today may be the one you'll want to explore in the future.

MADE FOR EACH OTHER: YOU AND YOUR HEALER

The process of selecting complementary practitioners is very similar to that of choosing therapies; you research and network, gathering as much information as you feel you need to make a choice—but with an added intensity, because you want to find exactly the right healer.

The way you experience any complementary therapy depends highly upon how it is administered and by whom. Whereas conventional medical treatment is often practiced in a fairly standard way, and sometimes offered on a rather impersonal level, working with a complementary healer is usually more varied. It's not like being treated for strep throat, where you receive a standard clinical evaluation, a prescription for antibiotics, and go home. Complementary practitioners work with you on a more intimate level, making the *way* treatment is given as important as the treatment itself. The practitioner becomes your healing partner, connecting with you on deeper levels to guide you through the healing that needs to take place. Complementary providers can offer rich, meaningful experiences that may be emotionally powerful and spiritually enlightening. They may serve as witnesses to significant growth on deeply personal issues. That is why selecting a complementary practitioner should be done as carefully as choosing a best friend. Complementary practitioners approach their practice with individual styles that often reflect a combination of their philosophy, training, and personality. Your success in part depends on your level of trust in and receptivity to the healers with whom you choose to work.

This is a new experience for many of us. We're used to

having our health care providers selected either through our health plans, by default when we seek care through a health clinic or local hospital, or by using the "if it's good enough for them, it's good enough for me" approach of adopting friends' or family members' choices. Because of this, you may feel uncomfortable taking full responsibility and making your selection autonomously.

Searching for healers can often feel like feast or famine. Either the possibilities seem limitless, or there just seems to be no one in your area. In both cases you will be left with your imagination, intuition, and inspiration to find who is out there for you. But whether you feel ready or not, you are better equipped than you think.

Hiring Your Healers

While several sources for finding healers are contained in the Appendix and Modalities sections, often the most abundant and easily accessible source will be the networking system that you have established. According to other survivors, the best advice is from those who have been there. Again, be relentless in your search; ask everyone you know for recommendations, particularly cancer survivors, people you know with experience in complementary treatments, and your own health team. You may want to ask your oncologist to put you in touch with other patients they know who are using complementary medicine; often they can be the ones you need to get started.

I was very fortunate to find a cancer survivor who was also a healer. She was extremely generous in serving as a mentor, leading me to colleagues she recommended and coaching me on hiring healers and selecting therapies. Now I coach others on creating integrative plans and selecting treatments and practitioners. More and more, coaches are becoming available for help in making complementary cancer choices. One survivor advises working with a coach and paying attention to the local scene. "Once you have healers you can trust, they can lead you to others and be a good source of information and guidance for your healing."

Listen for healers whose names come up repeatedly. Even in larger urban areas, the world of complementary practitioners is usually a fairly close-knit and supportive group. If you have access to local alternative health publications, organizations, or businesses, you may find they can be of help to you. Popular and effective practitioners in your community will be mentioned repeatedly. Your initial contact may not be your first choice for care, but don't stop there; keep asking for names, and you will get what you need.

SHOPPING TIP NO. 3:

Investigate the Practitioner as Much as the Practice

You may already have particular preferences regarding complementary practitioners, such as gender, medical background, survivor status, or the proximity of the practice. On the other hand, perhaps you are starting your search with *no* clear sense of what might work best for you. Wherever you begin, you will benefit by interviewing potential healers.

Interviewing healers may feel awkward at first, but it is invaluable in trying to ensure your success. Healers can make you more comfortable with a modality, clarify attitudes and expectations, and build confidence in your plan. You will find that most providers are very willing to be interviewed and generous with their time in explaining their work. If you come to them openly and honestly, they will meet you more than halfway.

I found interviewing healers to be a wonderful experience, since it helped establish good working relationships from the start. This in turn affected my interactions with *all* my caregivers. I became clearer and more outspoken about my expectations and needs, working with them more as a partner and less as a patient. Through interviewing, I found healers who empathized with my situation and did not condemn it, who saw my disease as a manifestation of my need to heal at deeper levels. I chose people who didn't announce they could fix me, but who said clearly what they could and couldn't provide. I listened for those healers who respected my decisions regarding conventional treatment and who were willing to work with them. By doing so, I was able to chose people who guided me faithfully through treatment and recovery.

SHOPPING TIP NO. 4:

Now, Take a Test Drive

You can conduct interviews by telephone, introducing yourself by briefly describing your cancer diagnosis and treatment plan. I did this not only to set the tone and make a connection with practitioners, but to get their reaction to my planned course of treatment; if they could not support my decisions, I wouldn't be able to work with them. I also explained why I was interested in working with their modality, and asked them if they had any reservations about me as a cancer patient. The following questions helped me to discern if there might be a good fit with a particular healer. Feel free to pick and choose from the chart, or compose your own questions. As you interview practitioners, try to pay attention not only to the answers, but also the feelings they evoke. Of course it works best to weave the questions into the conversation and avoid a "third degree" approach, which can alienate your practitioner and sabotage your goal of forming a strong partnership.

QUESTIONS FOR INTERVIEWING HEALERS

TREATMENT

- Can you describe how your therapy works?
- What does your type of treatment offer a person physically, emotionally, and spiritually? Do you have any data that would support this? Would you be willing to share it?
- Do you offer other forms of treatment? What are they, and would I benefit from them?
- What can I expect to feel from the treatments, both during and after, physically and emotionally? Are there common side effects? If so, what are they and how long do they last?

COMPATIBILITY

- How do you feel about conventional cancer treatment? How do you expect my cancer and/or my medical treatments to affect the process or outcome of our work together?
- Would interruption of our work because of medical complications (hospitalizations, treatment, disease side effects) cause a problem? Would you be able to come to me if I were ill?

EXPERIENCE

- What led you to your profession?
- What is your training? How does it compare with other programs in your field? How do you stay current in your field?
- Is your profession/modality licensed or certified in this state? Nationally?
- Are you licensed/certified?
- How long have you been in practice? How long in this area?

- Have you had experience with cancer patients?
- How do you feel about working with cancer?
- Do you feel the work you do helps people dealing with cancer? How?
- Would you be comfortable contacting any of your cancer patients who might be willing to talk to me about their experience?
- Would you be willing to give me names of your colleagues whom I might call as a reference?
- Do you have any experience working with physicians? Would you be open to working with mine, or with other members of my health team?
- Would you be willing to refer me, if needed, to other healers?

PRACTICE PARAMETERS
- Do you have an intake form? Do you keep session notes?
- Is there an expected/required or average length of treatment duration (i.e., number of sessions and length of each session)? *(This is useful if you are currently in treatment, and already have significant demands on your schedule because of treatments or side effects.)*
- Do you ever offer a "trial period" in which clients receive treatment for a limited number of sessions and then assess with you whether to continue?
- What are your treatment fees? Are there additional costs for such things as supplements, herbs, or additional therapies?
- Do you work with any insurance plans? Are you open to flexible financing?

WARNING: *Buyer beware! The insurance industry currently is in a particularly dynamic and sensitive state of flux with regard to coverage for complementary and alternative medicine. Determining coverage for complementary therapies can be extremely confusing for both practitioner and patient. Approach questions about insurance with caution, as what may be a legitimate answer can turn out to be erroneous information. You'll need to take responsibility for finding out what is true in your particular case.*

Don't be afraid to ask any questions you think of. You are forming a relationship on a very intimate level with this person, and you need to feel confident about your choice and to trust him or her. But a partnership *is* formed from the very beginning, and the more up front you can be with your needs and concerns, the better the practitioner will be able to serve you, right from the start.

LOSE YOUR MIND (AND COME TO YOUR SENSES)

After all the investigation and analysis, there is still that seemingly huge leap of faith to be made with your feelings. You have done your best to become an informed consumer, approaching the subject cautiously and educating yourself. But treatment decisions require using both sides of your brain. Take the time to pull together your feelings about the treatments you have studied and healers you've identified. Whether you are crystal clear about what you need to do or you feel conflicted, give yourself some space and solitude to go inside yourself and see what is taking shape. Ask yourself: Does the treatment seem helpful? Would it support one or more of my goals? Do I have any concerns that the treatment might hurt me? Are there questions left unanswered by the research I've done? Am I comfortable with leaving them unanswered? Weigh the information from your research with the goals and limitations you identified in Chapter 3. Have they changed because of what you have found in your research? If they have, it may indicate that you want to try the treatment regardless of your doubts.

Just as when you are choosing treatments (and, for that matter, physicians), you must tap your intuitive resources in making your practitioner selections. Someone may look good on paper, but if you don't feel right about him or her, chances are there's a good reason. While interviewing them, take note of how healers respond to your questions. Are they enthusiastic about their work? Do they describe their work and themselves in a way you can understand? Are they thoughtful and open to your needs? Are they willing to work as part of a larger team of healers? Do they appear to be well grounded, experienced, and dedicated? Are they defensive or does any answer make you uncomfortable? In other words, do they seem like people you can work with and trust to act on your best behalf?

If you are impressed with a healer who is not experienced working with cancer patients, that shouldn't necessarily stop you. Most healers do not base their approach solely on the particulars of their client's physical condition(s); rather they look at the whole person with individual needs, history, and current experience. Cancer is only one facet of the person, not the focus. If they have solid experience, are skilled in their profession, and have strong recommendations from colleagues or clients, then perhaps you are being called to work with them as part of the healing you need to do. You may want to check in with a trusted friend or health care practitioner and, of course, always inform and coordinate with your physician.

As you use intuition more and more in your decision-making, it will become increasingly clear where your heart wants to take you. And this may mean that you end up trying some treatments and healers that ultimately will be left behind. If you do, it doesn't mean that you can't trust your intuition; it just means the path can have some unexpected twists and turns. So try to lose your mind from time to time so you can listen to your heart. Allow yourself some space for trial and error, and forgive yourself for the detours. Intuition blossoms in the presence of patience and self-acceptance.

I was by no means an instant success in choosing the components of my plan. I had no idea what I was looking for in either therapies or healers when I started, but I sensed that I would know it when I found it. There was a lot of trial and error, but you do learn to tune into the right type of treatment and healer for you, so the process gets smoother with experience.

You are taking what feels like one tentative step at a time: finding a treatment, understanding it, selecting healers, and trying them out. You're feeling your way along as well as thinking it through as you approach your healing and choose your methods. Like any new journey, it can be exciting and frightening, sometimes tedious, and often frustrating. If you can live your intention, and return to your truth over and over in order to pursue the best path for *you*, it can be infinitely rewarding.

CHAPTER 5

LIVING YOUR PROMISE:
Making Your Plan Successful

*"In times of deepest despair, trust is offered to us
as well as asked of us."*

MAUREEN REDL, FOUNDER AND PRESIDENT, VOICES OF HEALING

If I could give you a recipe for success in developing your healing plan, it would look something like this:

- Two parts knowing yourself
- Three parts hard work
- Trust, as needed.

Knowing yourself is going inward and gaining a better understanding of what you feel to be your truth. Through knowing yourself, you are loving yourself more, making a deeper connection with the Divine, and counting on yourself to live out your truth, your promise. It's the embodiment of trust.

While it may sound as though trust is thrown into the recipe as an afterthought, it really is the key component of healing. All the research, interviewing, and decision-making connected to your healing plan is, of course, based on trust—of your capabilities and the help that is sent your way. And living your plan requires a deep and sustaining trust, respecting the mystery of healing without perhaps understanding it at all.

Trying to embrace trust fully can be a challenging task. It requires a vulnerability that can be particularly difficult when you are already feeling laid open by the disease. Trust can be undefinable and hard to quantify or qualify, if you can do it at all. It's only natural, though, to want to assess where we are in our process as we strive to heal ourselves. We want to come to know the depth of our trust, as well as what we need to do with that trust.

Three attributes help us to better trust, understand, and accept. These attributes are at the root of any healing plan and are critical to its success; they will feed your actions, strengthen your decision-making, and carry you through any setbacks.

Confidence is about caring for yourself more by manifesting your inner wisdom through life-affirming action. *Commitment* means counting on yourself to see it through and drawing upon your love for yourself and what you receive from others for support. *Communication* involves opening up to your inner dialogue, trusting what you find inside, and expressing that self-trust to others, in order to realize your goals and respect your process.

These attributes are interdependent, forming a delicate, fluctuating balance. As one wanes, you will find you need to call upon the others for reinforcement. I haven't seen any healing plan that doesn't contain them.

Confidence, commitment, and communication: why do you need them? Because they will be the foundation that will support your healing and help you live your promise. But how do you get them, and how can you keep them?

CONFIDENCE

Most survivors I know, including myself, have had to talk their way into feeling confident about their complementary treatment choices. After all, cancer betrays us. You may feel robbed of any faith in your ability to heal and to monitor your body's needs and state of health. So why would you trust that you could be in charge of your healing by using treatments that, in our culture, appear to be unproven and "on the edge"?

Developing an integrated treatment plan is no small undertaking, and there may be times when you are immobilized by the task. That's when you most need confidence, to nudge you out of that space and move you into action. You don't have to create enthusiasm out of thin air for each treatment or practitioner you try, convinced that this is "the one." That's unrealistic, puts unnecessary stress on you, and sets you up for disappointment. Rather, what's needed here is an underlying belief that you are on track, and that if you veer off course, you will be guided back. Confidence is both a deep knowledge that your intention is right, and an opening to that knowledge in order to motivate you and remove the doubts when they come. Confidence brings with it an objective curiosity to try what you believe will help. And if it doesn't, confidence gives you faith that the experience will bring you to what's necessary to heal. Confidence can prepare and sustain you for all the work and growth ahead.

Gaining and keeping confidence comes over time and through positive experiences with your plan. It is planted through clarifying your expectations of complementary care and being honest about your limitations. It grows through doing your homework: researching, networking, observing other survivors' experiences. And it is nurtured by living in the present moment. So many of us try to stay one step ahead of the future: reading every new book, following every lead, expending energy on research of cutting-edge treatments and promising therapies we may need someday. But doing this puts us in a "no-win" situation because it never ends. We sabotage ourselves because it keeps us from being where we need to be: with ourselves, in the present. By giving ourselves that sacred space, we give ourselves a gift, a way to gain clarity and truly know what our future needs to be. We live our promise.

Confidence thrives on commitment and communication with yourself, wherever you may be in your healing. "Confiding" is at the heart of confidence. Reaching new levels of honesty with yourself can be very difficult to achieve, but it is essential. The intentions behind all your actions stem from self-revelation. If you are able to confide in yourself *about* yourself thoroughly and openly, then you will know your needs clearly enough to manifest them. Confidence will flourish when you trust your intuition.

COMMITMENT

Your integrated treatment plan can be viewed as a critical tool to be used only during cancer treatment and recovery, or it can be a lifestyle change, a permanent asset in your life. Either way, it calls for commitment.

You are beginning a beautifully creative process, which in itself ignites and nourishes your life force. While the basic goal of healing stays constant, the style and substance of your path offer endless possibilities. In building the best environment for your health, you need to give yourself over to it totally.

Commitment is essential because healing is an open-ended process, lasting as long as you wish. Healing from cancer can serve as a catalyst for continual expansion, making it a wondrous, illuminating experience. But it can also demand huge investments of time and energy, challenging you at the deepest level to stay with it through the trials and errors and continual fine tuning. Throughout your healing, you will see your commitment ebb and flow like the tides. You may question your commitment, lose it, cling to it, and strengthen it over and over again. The cyclical nature of commitment is natural, allowing your healing to take place exactly as it needs to. But this ebb and flow can be frightening for many. Using complementary therapies is often a dance between blind faith and logic.

How do you commit yourself to integrative healing? By having patience and developing flexibility and perseverance. You are in the process of learning a new way to listen to your body and how it heals. You will be better able to recognize how and when your needs change at different stages of healing. I had to learn to trust my body's knowledge and honor my intuition; knowing when to stop a treatment was as important as knowing when to start. I began to view stopping a therapy not as a sign of failure, but as a sign that my body was moving toward a different level of healing. I no longer saw my healers as separate entities, but as a healing team, with a tremendous mix of skills that I could draw upon when needed. And finally I began to understand that healing reveals itself over time, not as human beings mark it, but in universal time. If you can learn to trust this gradual revelation, then you are better able to commit to the process.

Staying committed can be fostered by becoming part of the community that uses complementary treatment for cancer. By choosing to explore complementary therapies, you are introduced to a powerful, supportive community of fellow survivors and healers that can help keep you focused. Know, too, that as you help them with their confidence and commitment to healing, you help yourself as well.

It's also important to be clear about the level of commitment made by your physicians and complementary practitioners. It helps to know whether there is mutual commitment and where it exists. For instance, soon after beginning to work with the surgeon who diagnosed me, I sensed a great sadness whenever he saw me. I realized that he truly believed there was no hope for my recovery. When I discovered that he wasn't committed to my healing, I could no longer work with him. Surround yourself with people who are truly aligned with your intentions; you need to know where you are *both* committed. From that common spark you can draw from the fire of shared commitment—and call upon the other's commitment when yours wanes.

Commitment involves visiting the past, staying in the present, and looking to the future simultaneously. Look back at where you were just before you were diagnosed, acknowledging how the changes you have made since then have helped you. Feel where you are *now*: what your body, spirit, and psyche need at this moment. Realize that by doing so, you are becoming more sensitive and attuned to your needs, consciously staying with the healing process despite any self-doubt or fear. You are living your commitment! And look ahead, visualizing the way you want to be, the freedoms you desire, and the unfolding of yourself that's waiting for you. It will help you to stay the course.

COMMUNICATION

Communication completes the plan's foundation as the bridge between the other attributes. It helps you to access support when your confidence is flagging. It affirms your commitment through sharing your needs and goals, and facilitates your meeting them. Having a successful integrated treatment plan does not allow you to work in a vacuum or be shrouded in secrecy. Rather, it calls you to interact on a more intimate level with all who care for you and about you. Establishing working relationships that allow full expression of needs and promote feedback will be an important part of your plan.

When discussing communication, the experience of cancer patients exploring complementary therapy is, in my mind, akin to that of adolescents exploring their sexuality. For both groups, examining these topics involves highly personal choices, is rife with misinformation, and fraught with risks—emotional, physical, and spiritual. It can also elicit harsh judgments from loved ones. In both cases, though, the desire to discover something for yourself burns brightly, and may result in a person "going underground." In the case of complementary treatment, it could mean a number of things, including accepting questionable recommendations or secretly combining multiple therapies that may compromise conventional treatments or your health. It's better to bring the whole process out into the light so that you can find people who can support you.

If you have family and friends willing to help, talk to them about your goals in using complementary therapies and the actual treatments you're using. By sharing your understanding of the roles of these therapies, your loved ones can be of tremendous value in helping you over the bumps when you are feeling frustrated. Elaine Callinan, a massage therapist who has worked with many cancer patients, has observed her clients struggling with a sense of isolation from family and friends as they use complementary therapies. "Sharing your plans, path, process, and experience with them will alleviate the helplessness and frustration they experience in their love for you. They *need* you to share how you're taking charge of your healing. This is where they can join you in your recovery—in your frustrations and progress."

Reach out to other survivors; communicate your desire to find support within the cancer community for your healing plan. You can find camaraderie in talking with other survivors. And you may discover that your common experiences can nurture your confidence and strengthen your commitment.

Communication with Complementary Practitioners
Of course it's crucial to be able to communicate with your practitioners. One of the main benefits in doing this

work is assembling a team of healers. But to make that team successful, you must be able to discuss your needs clearly and coordinate your healing. I wouldn't have received what I did from my healing without open relationships with my healers. I had to learn to share my disappointments and fears, to feel comfortable asking questions and expressing doubts and feelings. When I felt the need to move on, I had to acknowledge my need and end my work with that practitioner.

This kind of communication can be quite different from what we have previously experienced. I was far from accustomed to being in partnership with practitioners and responsible for directing my health care. But I found that practicing open communication placed the relationship with my healers in a better balance. My feelings and intuition were respected and incorporated into my treatment. Many healers whom I've interviewed have expressed gratitude for their relationships with cancer clients, for what they have received from them, and for the new ways they have incorporated what they have learned into their practice. Such open partnerships can extend beyond the two participants, affecting the whole community of healers and survivors.

Communication with Physicians

Communication as a cornerstone of your integrated treatment plan will inevitably influence your relationships with your medical team, hopefully in a positive way. We have already discussed the difficulties encountered by many survivors in sharing their treatment plans with their physicians, but I emphasize the need to keep your doctors informed of all you are doing to help yourself heal. If you are under a doctor's care and concurrently undergoing complementary treatment, you are only sabotaging yourself in keeping the two separate, adding to your stress, and undermining your relationship with your doctor.

Open communication with your physician can offer you a better relationship overall. As I worked with my complementary healers, I gained the confidence I needed to approach my doctors in the same way and found myself being much more up front about my needs and wants in general. I demanded better explanations of treatment protocols and decisions and was able to convey the degree of involvement I wished to have in my care. I learned what I could about my condition, so that I could be more involved in discussing treatment options and better manage my illness. It leveled the field for me and my doctors, and gave all of us the opportunity to make the doctor-patient relationship more healthy and whole.

In part I credit open communication with my medical team's ability to support my use of complementary treatment, for which I was very grateful. For instance, by keeping my team informed of my desire to continue with my complementary regimen during my bone marrow treatment, they were able to facilitate the use of many of my modalities during my long-term hospitalization. Knowledge of my integrative plan also led my doctors to share my progress with other patients eager to talk with fellow survivors about complementary therapies. Open communication fostered mutual trust and respect for our individual decisions on the course of my care.

Communicating in the wake of negative feedback from your physician is obviously more of a challenge, but it is necessary to maintain the integrity of your intention. Explain the benefits of your complementary treatment and the impact that his or her opinion has on it. It will help you to clarify the value you place on complementary care, and whether you have the support you need to truly heal. It can also strengthen your commitment to your integrated treatment plan, and lead you to make changes in your medical care that will make it more harmonious with your integrative approach.

If you have the good fortune to find a doctor who embraces the use of complementary treatments or shows an interest in these practices, I would urge you to support your doctor's growth in this area as much as possible. Provide her or him with additional knowledge and encourage involvement with your complementary healers. They need to see the results of integrative healing, not be sheltered from it. We need to encourage them to respond not only to their patients seeking complementary care, but to incorporate such therapies, if possible, as treatment options or adjunct therapies for others who may not be aware such treatments exist.

You owe it to yourself to be forthcoming about your choices with *all* your caregivers if your goal is truly to integrate your care. Let your oncologists know when you have added or stopped using a particular treatment. They may show interest, offer a new perspective, or ask you to explain or defend your position. But they need to know in order to serve you better. It's not an integrated treatment plan if your doctors have no knowledge of your complementary healers! If you feel the need to maintain the distinction between complementary and conventional care, be alert to the ways the separation affects your confidence and commitment to your plan.

LIVING YOUR PLAN

Cancer deserves a second look. For all of us, it comes packaged as a crisis, a threat, a possible ending. But if you look again, you can find incredible opportunities, new beginnings, courage, and love unlike anything you have ever experienced. Cancer awakens your consciousness, grants you wisdom, and heightens your senses. It reconnects you to life with blinding speed and intensity and demands acknowledgment and acceptance of your passions. It teaches you to love yourself and come to terms with humanity.

Creating an integrated treatment plan forces you to engage more fully in the cancer experience, to go beyond the physical level. It is a powerful act of self-affirmation that enables you to make a deeper commitment to loving yourself. Your plan is your promise, your gift; it brings you face to face with cancer's offer to define living for yourself. To design your plan without living it would be to turn away from yourself, when what you need more than anything is to find yourself.

For me, living my plan meant allowing myself to be surrounded by dedicated, talented professionals who devoted themselves to supporting me through treatments and recovery at a personal, meaningful level. It meant approaching life in a new way, looking at new experiences as contributing to my healing, regardless of how they were packaged. Through my adjustment, for instance, I found myself able to receive spiritual support from my allopathic team instead of just girding myself for the difficult physical treatments. By opening up to these new perspectives, my plan began to weave itself together.

Living my plan also meant discovering how to nurture myself, which allowed me to love myself more genuinely. This in turn opened me up to others in a more honest and generous way.

And living my plan required decision-making from the heart, which touched all aspects of my life and helped me to heal from more than just my disease. It helped me to find my faith. Consciously participating in my healing brought to me wonder and joy, which I'd never expected to find in this process. It helped me to express deep gratitude for our time here and to trust in the Divine. And it showed me that you can survive cancer and flourish, whether it's in mending relationships, teaching others, living life more fully, or finding God. It's all in how you live your promise: how you create it and how you allow yourself to accept it. What incredible gifts I have received! Eight years after my initial cancer diagnosis, I am still in awe of the experience and of each day I am given in which to receive more of life.

Ellen Grayson, a dear friend and fellow survivor told me, "You have the right to *all* these gifts." That is a message for all of us. I couldn't agree with her more.

I hope you do, too.

PART II
COMPLEMENTARY
HEALING THERAPIES

TREATMENT MODALITIES
Introduction

The modalities described here were selected because of their popularity, availability, and efficacy in supporting healing from cancer. These selections were based on conversations with other survivors experienced in using complementary therapy, the advice of complementary practitioners and health care professionals, and my personal experience as well as that of Dr. Rick Steinberg, a physician and cancer survivor who assisted with this book.

These modalities were carefully selected to include a broad spectrum of therapies that support all phases of healing: physical, mental, emotional, and spiritual. Cancer survivors have attested to their aiding the healing process. No one treatment is recommended over another, nor are they all-inclusive. Many roads lead to the same destination.

The descriptions of each modality, therefore, are meant to serve as introductions to selected complementary therapies, providing a starting point from which to explore these therapies and investigate others on your own. There are as many ways to classify these modalities as there are therapies. In this case, I have grouped several within larger categories, while some stand alone.

I have intentionally made the modality descriptions brief, for two reasons. First, life with cancer is overwhelming enough: I did not want to weigh down the book (and you) with lengthy descriptions. Second, there are already some excellent resources that provide as much information as you could want; I saw no need to reinvent them. But I did feel that it would be unfair to advise you on developing an integrated treatment plan without giving you a place to start.

Each description includes a brief overview of each therapy, a discussion of how the therapies are beneficial to cancer patients, and a description of the treatment experience. You will also find interviews with many creative, skilled providers, with expertise in each of the featured modalities. These interviews provide personal accounts of how these therapies are applied to the cancer experience, and illustrate the variety of approaches used in complementary cancer care. They also serve as examples of how the tools provided earlier in this book can be applied. Introducing you to these professionals and allowing them to describe their work provides you an opportunity to better understand what complementary cancer care is and the variety of ways it can be delivered.

The chapters also include information on training and professional credentials. Understanding training, credentialing, and licensing requirements can be complicated and confusing because rules and procedures vary by profession and from state to state. However, it's a good idea to familiarize yourself with training and professional standards for modalities you pursue, since complementary care remains largely underregulated.

Two additional sections are included in each modality. "For Further Information" identifies organizations where you can obtain information on the profession. Many of these organizations provide research databases that you can access. Often, these organizations will provide practitioner referrals. Their requirements for listing practitioners vary broadly and are worth a little investigation. Listings may consist of their entire membership; some represent healers who have taken only one course or perhaps completed a program from their organization; still others may have been required to meet specific, more rigorous eligibility criteria. Listed practitioners are not necessarily endorsed by the providing organization. You may wish to consult with the organizations directly for further information and assistance. (Please note that while public requests are welcome, most of these organizations are not equipped to deal with individual telephone inquiries. If at all possible, access their web site first.)

Finally, the "Books Recommended by Healers" section lists additional references suggested by practitioners and other health professionals interviewed for this book.

Three reference resources I have relied upon for my own healing, and for the compilation of the modality descriptions, are:

- *Alternative Medicine: The Definitive Guide.* Compiled by The Burton Goldberg Group (Fife, Washington: Future Medicine Publishing Group, 1993)
- *The Best Alternative Medicine: What Works? What Does Not?* Kenneth Pelletier, M.D. (New York: Simon and Schuster, 2000)
- *The Alternative Medicine Handbook: The Complete Guide to Alternative and Complementary Therapies.* Barrie Cassileth, Ph.D. (New York: W.W. Norton and Company, 1998)

These are excellent representatives of the many fine resource guides on complementary therapies. I highly recommend that you obtain one or two guides for your personal library. Many thanks to these authors for providing such comprehensive, detailed, and balanced guides.

A book I consider to be essential reading for those considering or already using complementary therapy for cancer is Michael Lerner's wonderful book *Choices in Healing: Integrating the Best of Conventional and Complementary Approaches to Cancer* (Cambridge, Massachusetts: The MIT Press, 1994). It presents a conscientious overview of complementary and conventional therapies and guides the reader with insight and caring through several modalities. This is a beautifully written book that gives comfort and trustworthy knowledge. It can be found on-line in its entirety at www.commonweal.org/choicescontents.html.

Finally, every effort has been made to provide current information on the modalities. However, because the field of complementary therapy is fluid, new data and discoveries have the potential to impact the timeliness of the information presented here. I would encourage you to try to stay current with any modalities that are of interest to you, and to update your resources on a regular basis.

A NOTE FROM THE AUTHOR

I received an unexpected education in my research for this section of the book. Part of my motivation for producing this book was based on wanting to share what I believed was my own considerable knowledge of complementary therapies, which I had gained through my own personal experience and through coaching others. But as I attempted to write clear, concise, and accurate descriptions of these modalities, my eyes were further opened to the dynamics—and complexity—of integrative medicine, particularly within the context of conventional cancer care.

What I found is that each modality selected for this book seems to be in its own phase of evolution. Some modalities are in the process of establishing themselves as formal disciplines or professions. For example, experts in the fields are attempting to establish training and credentialing standards, acquiring insurance reimbursement, and so on. Naturally, these are somewhat easier to qualify. Other modalities, however, are still in the process of defining their relationship to our cultural conception of health and illness, or determining their role in integrative medicine. As such, they can appear to be unstructured or vague.

While I have strived to present an accurate picture of each modality, the dynamic nature of complementary therapy has made it particularly challenging. As I consulted references, conferred with healers, and received reviewers' comments, I was struck by the speed at which information changes, the lack of a unified, authoritative voice, and the levels of passion found in conflicting philosophies and opinions.

Through sifting and sorting the information I collected, I have come to appreciate even more the treasure we have in accessing our inner wisdom when forming our individual healing plans and determining our choices. Ideologies differ. Training, experience, and the skill levels of practitioners vary. The effectiveness of different treatments can be subjective. All can impact your care. Many authors warn of the risks associated with complementary therapy, and urge people to proceed with caution and with "eyes wide open." While I can agree with their caution to some extent—particularly when dealing with cancer—I believe it's just as important, if not more so, to go in with your heart wide open.

With the variety of choices we have, I urge caution from the standpoint of finding the best care possible for *you*, which means using both sides of your brain and then some. I view the challenge of cancer treatment not as black or white, as abandoning one form of treatment for the other. Rather, I hope you will explore what you find —whether conventional or complementary—to the best of your ability. Question not just with your mind, but with your heart, and feel as much as you think your way through your options. In other words, put your whole self *into* your healing decisions, so you can get your whole self *back*.

ACUPUNCTURE

Many Western physicians now offer acupuncture, a major component of traditional Chinese medicine, as part of their practices. Studies have reported that acupuncture can help relieve some types of pain, and also reduce nausea and other side effects from conventional cancer treatments.

According to traditional Chinese medicine, acupuncture, a centuries-old system of healing, helps balance qi (pronounced "chee"), the vitality, or "life energy," that belongs to all living things. Qi is believed to flow along meridians, energy pathways that course throughout the body. The meridians interconnect and support the delivery of qi to all organs and muscles.

Qi deficiency or stagnation anywhere in the body is thought to inhibit healing and increase discomfort. By balancing qi in the body, acupuncture helps maintain or restore our overall health and functioning.

Acupuncture treatment largely consists of using extremely small, sterile, disposable stainless steel needles (no thicker than a human hair), which are inserted at specific acupuncture points along the meridians. In the traditional view, the insertion of the needles stimulates or redirects the flow of qi. This restores balance to the life force and improves overall health.

There are several different kinds of acupuncture. For instance, in traditional Chinese medicine, practitioners provide herbal treatments along with the use of needles.

Medical acupuncture, which is practiced by medical doctors and osteopathic physicians, often integrates Western medicine with Chinese treatments. Another type of acupuncture, called auricular acupuncture, focuses on the manipulation of acupuncture points of the ear.

■ HOW IT HELPS ■

In the traditional view, acupuncture is an integral part of whole-body wellness. When qi is balanced, energy flows smoothly through the body, without blockages. Practitioners believe that when all of the body's muscles, organs, and other systems receive the appropriate amounts of qi, illnesses, including cancer, are less likely to occur.

In the last few decades, scientists in the West have begun to investigate the use of acupuncture for easing the discomfort caused by conventional cancer treatments. Acupuncture has been found to be helpful in reducing side effects from surgery, chemotherapy, or radiation treatments, such as nausea, certain types of pain (musculoskeletal pain, for example), and fatigue. "Acupuncture addresses some of the side effects of chemotherapy and radiation therapy by helping to restore improved function to stressed organs," says Robert Shapero, M.Ac., L.Ac., a licensed acupuncturist at Acupuncture Family Health Services in Bethesda, Maryland.

In one study, 104 women undergoing high-dose chemotherapy were treated either with antinausea drugs alone or with drugs plus electroacupuncture, a technique in which electrical pulses are transmitted through the acupuncture needles. Those who received the acupuncture treatments experienced less discomfort than those who were given medications alone. Over five days of treatment, women in the acupuncture group had less than half the episodes of nausea and vomiting than those in the drug-only group.[9]

Another common use of acupuncture by cancer patients is to relieve pain. Doctors theorize that the insertion of needles stimulates the nervous system to release morphine-like chemicals called endorphins. Acupuncture shouldn't be used as a replacement for conventional medical treatment in easing cancer pain—the pain that occurs when a tumor presses against nerves or other tissues—because it has not been found to be particularly effective as a substitute for pain-killing drugs in this instance. But it can be a helpful adjunct to opioid medications. For instance, some doctors are combining acupuncture and conventional pain medication to control surgery-related pain, and in some cases acupuncture can reduce the need for pain medication. In addition, acupuncture has been reported to be useful for other types of pain that many cancer patients face, such as the pain from headache, arthritis, and other musculoskeletal conditions.

Both Eastern and Western practitioners of acupuncture believe that acupuncture can be effective in stimulating immune function. Acupuncture has been shown to be effective in increasing the number of white blood cells and T-cells in HIV and AIDS patients. An increase in white blood cells is important because it stimulates the body's defensive abilities to fend off infection and heal more quickly.

Because acupuncture can increase energy and promote feelings of well-being, it may help give people the inner strength they need to undergo necessary cancer treatments. Many cancer patients report that side effects from treatments are more difficult to cope with than the illness itself. "Chinese medicine successfully affects our emotional balance; it can lift a person's spirits or calm someone's anxiety, if needed," says Shapero.

Cancer patients who incorporate acupuncture in their overall treatment plans report they sleep better at night, have improved appetite and digestion, and generally feel stronger.

■ WHAT TO EXPECT ■

If you decide to incorporate acupuncture into a cancer treatment plan, keep in mind that it's an on-going process. Studies suggest that while acupuncture can provide significant relief from pain, nausea, and other side effects of treatment, patients may require repeated visits. Some people make weekly acupuncture appointments; others get the treatments only after surgery; others throughout radiation or chemotherapy treatments.

When you see an acupuncturist, the treatment usually begins with a detailed medical history. A physical examination is done, with particular focus on the tongue and pulse, both considered indicators of health and disease. The pulse is taken on the radial artery at varying depths on each wrist, to ascertain the condition of the organs and the flow of qi through the meridians. Also taken into account are skin color, urine color, voice tone, and tolerance of heat and cold, all of which are believed to contribute to an accurate picture of the patient's health.

An acupuncture treatment may be given during the first session. Based on the acupuncturist's examination and diagnosis, specific acupuncture points are selected to facilitate the redirection of energy. The needles are inserted just under the skin, usually in no more than ten to twelve sites. The needles may be twirled slightly to enhance their effectiveness. For most people the procedure is painless. Some people feel a slight prick, and others report feelings of heaviness, tingling, heat, or mild tugging, that quickly dissipate.

Needles are usually left in place for no more than thirty minutes. Many patients feel relaxed and may fall asleep during treatment. Chronic conditions may call for a series of regular treatments, usually given weekly. It is not uncommon to schedule regular acupuncture appointments throughout the year as part of routine health care.

Acupuncturists use a variety of techniques. These include electrostimulation of acupuncture points, or the application of laser beams or ultrasound. Moxibustion is the application of a heated herb, mugwort, directly above an acupuncture point. Cupping is another procedure practiced by some acupuncturists. Air is heated inside glass cups, which are then placed on acupuncture points or on painful areas to create suction. The treatment is believed to help circulation and qi movement.

■ TRAINING ■

The National Certification Council for Acupuncture and Oriental Medicine (NCCAOM) certifies three distinct types of practitioners: acupuncturist, Chinese herbalist, and oriental bodywork therapist. The NCCAOM-approved acupuncture training is a full-time three-year program (1,725 training hours). There are approximately fifty approved training programs in the United States. (Note: There are other non–NCCAOM-certified acupuncture training programs, some of which are less extensive.)

Medical doctors and physicians have their own training program, with more emphasis on integrating Chinese medicine with Western medicine, which follows their medical education. Their certification is obtained through the American Academy of Medical Acupuncture (AAMA). The AAMA is a professional society of physicians (both M.D.s and D.O.s) who have post–medical school training in acupuncture and have incorporated acupuncture into their traditional Western medical practice. AAMA certification requirements include 300 hours of training, two years of clinical experience, and successful completion of a written examination.

As of 1999, thirty-four states use NCCAOM as their acupuncture licensure protocol. In some states NCCAOM certification is the only criteria for licensure; others have set additional criteria.

Thirty-eight states and the District of Columbia currently regulate acupuncture; other states have legislation pending. Some states require licensure; others certification or registration. In a few states, acupuncture licensure is granted to M.D. applicants based primarily on their medical degree rather than certified acupuncture training. It's important to find out how your state regulates acupuncture.

Health insurance coverage for acupuncture varies by state and insurance company.

■ TREATMENTS FROM TOP PRACTITIONERS ■

Robert Heffron, M.D., *is a physician and medical acupuncturist in Providence, Rhode Island. He practices traditional, complementary, and oriental medicine. He estimates that approximately ten percent of his patients are living with cancer.*

Treatment Goals

With training in internal medicine, Chinese medicine, nutrition, and osteopathic manipulation, Dr. Heffron utilizes tools from many disciplines in his work with cancer patients.

He often takes advantage of acupuncture and other techniques from Chinese medicine because he feels they can help people move toward a greater awareness of disease-causing as well as health-promoting behaviors.

"Chinese medicine is one of the most comprehensive medical systems," says Dr. Heffron. "It incorporates the energetic and physical aspects of our being, and it respects individuality—which is important because all diseases are uniquely manifested by each person. Chinese medicine has the tools to understand a patient's past history and present condition, as well as to intervene in processes that may contribute to future illness."

Treatment Session

Early sessions are oriented toward patient and practitioner finding a way to connect on a deep level. An initial visit is approximately ninety minutes long and is used to record a comprehensive health history.

The next session lasts seventy-five minutes. Additional information is taken about the patient's history, and the session also includes a physical exam, which focuses on the tongue, abdomen, and especially the pulse. Treatment may be initiated at this time, depending on the complexity of the problem.

Follow-up visits last seventy-five minutes, and usually include reevaluation, acupuncture, and herbal prescriptions. Dr. Heffron's treatments may also include moxibustion, osteopathic manipulations, and counseling about health-related issues.

Patients often feel deeply relaxed following the treatments. In some cases, however, reactions to treatments don't fully unfold for up to seventy-two hours, says Dr. Heffron. Patients may feel an emotional or physical release, and they often feel uplifted. Adverse reactions—such as a small bruise where a needle was injected, or fatigue on the day of treatment—are rare.

Benefits to Cancer Patients

Dr. Heffron believes that cancer is a manifestation of internal disharmony. He uses acupuncture to help people tap into their own healing resources, often trying to help them let go and unravel emotional issues that impede them from healing and living a full life. He also uses herbs to support and build the immune system, as well as herbs that may directly affect cancerous cells.

Compatibility with Conventional Treatment

Dr. Heffron's approach to treatment is very compatible with conventional therapies. His patients usually work with an oncologist in conjunction with his treatments, and he often confers with other treating physicians.

■ ■ ■

Floyd Herdrich, M.Ac., L.Ac., *practices acupuncture in Bethesda, Maryland, and Falls Church, Virginia.*

Treatment Goals

"I don't heal patients," says Herdrich, "I help point the body in the right direction and the body heals itself. Acupuncture diagnosis is used to assess a person's energetic predisposition to compromises in their health. I use these diagnostic tools to place acupuncture needles in specific points to improve the balance and flow of energy that supports normal, healthy functions. This helps people to make shifts that allow them to be more resilient and to cope better. Acupuncture can improve the quality of patients' lives so that they are better able to live and be with their disease. Acupuncture patients' physicians have noted that their patients' recovery from treatment was faster than anticipated.

"I also offer Oriental Bodywork Therapy (OBT), known as Tui Na or medical massage in the Orient. OBT addresses patient ailments through conscious manipulation of the body and the qi body for restoring health."

Treatment Session

The initial session is a two-hour evaluation of a patient's life and health history. The next session is a two-hour treatment where acupuncture points are needled and responses are observed by checking pulses, color, odor, sound, and emotions. Often only one or two points are stimulated at one time, and re-evaluations and adjustments are made throughout the session. Subsequent sessions usually last one hour and begin with a brief re-evaluation, followed by an acupuncture treatment. "Generally people become more relaxed and refreshed during treatment. Often people describe themselves as feeling more open and in tune, better able to deal with whatever is affecting them. It helps people to let go of areas of stress and discomfort so that the body is better able to cope."

Benefits to Cancer Patients

In addition to the benefits already mentioned, Herdrich reports that acupuncture improves immune function, helps people to sleep better, and makes them generally more resilient. "There is also good evidence that it helps with side effects of chemotherapy and radiation such as fatigue and nausea."

Compatibility with Conventional Treatment

"Acupuncture is very compatible with conventional cancer treatment and contributes to patient recovery, well-being, and quality of life," says Herdrich. "Coordination with the patient's physician(s) is preferred. There are no problems of 'interaction' with prescribed treatments. Acupuncture treatment supports the natural health systems of the patient: it does not 'cure' the disease. Acupuncture may well support the natural defenses of the patient, which in turn may overcome the manifestation of cancer."

FOR FURTHER INFORMATION

A directory of NCCAOM-certified diplomates is available at the NCCAOM web site: www.nccaom.org, or by calling: (703) 548-9004. AAMA invites all of its members (currently over 1,900) to list themselves on the AAMA referral service for patients. About half of the membership is represented on the present list. For a copy, call (800) 521-2262, or visit www.medicalacupuncture.org.

The American Association of Oriental Medicine (AAOM), a professional membership organization representing licensed acupuncturists and students, provides a listing of state acupuncture associations and referrals to their members, who must meet specific eligibility criteria. Information on state associations and AAOM members can be obtained by calling (888) 500-7999. Their web site is www.aaom.org.

National Certification Commission for
Acupuncture and Oriental Medicine
11 Canal Center Plaza, Suite 300
Alexandria, VA 22314   (703) 548-9004

American Association of Oriental Medicine
5530 Wisconsin Avenue, Suite 1210
Chevy Chase, MD 20815   (301) 941-1064, (888) 500-7999

American Academy of Medical Acupuncture
4929 Wilshire Boulevard, Suite 428
Los Angeles, CA 90010   (323) 937-5514

BOOKS RECOMMENDED BY HEALERS

Between Heaven and Earth: A Guide to Chinese Medicine. Harriet Beinfield and Efrem Korngold (New York: Ballantine Books, 1991).

Restored Harmony: An Evidence-Based Approach for Integrating Traditional Chinese Medicine into Complementary Cancer Care. Stephen Sagar, M.D. (Hamilton, Ontario: Dreaming Dragonfly Communications, 2001).

The Web That Has No Weaver: Understanding Chinese Medicine. Ted J. Kaptchuk (Chicago: Congdon and Weed, 1983).

The comprehensive health system called Ayurveda has been practiced for over five thousand years, originating in India and gaining recent popularity in the United States. Ayurveda has been called a "whole-life" system because it addresses every aspect of the body, mind, and spirit. As such, it can be a valuable adjunct to mainstream cancer care. Many Ayurvedic therapies such as massage, yoga, meditation, and the use of medicinal herbs can complement conventional cancer treatments by helping to reduce stress, improve immunity, and reduce some of the side effects of cancer therapy such as nausea, fatigue, and muscle aches.

The philosophy of Ayurveda is based on the understanding that all living things are composed of three universal qualities called "doshas." These three doshas—vata, pitta, and kapha—govern all the biological, psychological, and physiological functions of the body, mind, and consciousness. One's individual constitution is acquired at birth and remains constant throughout life. The doshas represent combinations of the five elements: earth, air, fire, water, and ether. An interdependent relationship exists between the three doshas. In general, there are seven types of mind/body constitutions, created by dosha combinations, variation, and predominance. Among these seven types are innumerable subtle variations that depend upon the percentage of vata-pitta-kapha elements in one's constitution.

It is the proper balancing of the doshas that results in good health. Each person's mind/body type is believed to represent his or her physical, emotional, and spiritual constitution. When the doshas are out of balance, the body is more susceptible to stress and disease. Ayurvedic medicine relies upon long-held knowledge, the body's wisdom and natural composition, holistic practice, and the patient's commitment to self-care to maintain mental, physical, and spiritual health and well-being. "Most of the people with cancer I've seen are highly motivated to find out what they can do for themselves," adds Catherine K. Carson, D.C., C.Ad., an Ayurvedic practitioner at the Ayurveda Mind-Body Health Center in Fairfax, Virginia. "Among those who are highly motivated, I have seen some excellent results."

■ HOW IT HELPS ■

Because Ayurveda's goal is to detect and correct imbalance, it appears to be most beneficial in the promotion and maintenance of health. It emphasizes maintaining a healthy environment through improvements to a person's emotional, physical, and spiritual harmony. While Ayurveda's principles are best applied to preventing illness, they can be effective in supporting cancer patients, regardless of where they are in the treatment process. Patients often value Ayurveda for its calming, restorative, and rejuvenating effects.

As a preventive practice, Ayurveda focuses on strengthening the immune system, thereby enhancing a person's resistance to illness or environmental insults such as toxins in air, food, or water. Some aspects of Ayurveda appear to play specific roles in cancer prevention and in reducing fatigue and other side effects from conventional cancer therapy. One example is diet. The Ayurvedic diet is individualized, as every person requires different amounts and combinations of foods. It is interesting to note that despite the ancient origins of Ayurveda, many of the dietary recommendations are almost identical to those espoused by modern cancer researchers. Consider, for example, broccoli, cabbage, and Brussels sprouts: from an Ayurvedic standpoint, these are classified as "pungent" and "bitter" foods that pacify the Earth principle. In purely scientific terms, they're rich in isothiocyanates, chemical compounds that have been shown to block the harmful effects of cell-damaging toxins.

Most Ayurvedic practitioners recommend a vegetarian diet, although small amounts of fish are often included. For people with cancer, or for those who simply want to prevent it, a plant-based diet has many advantages. Whole grains, legumes, vegetables, and other plant foods are rich in phytochemicals, plant compounds that may stimulate the activity of immune cells, inhibit genetic mutations, and neutralize environmental toxins. Many phytochemicals act as antioxidants, blocking the action of harmful oxygen molecules known as free radicals on the body, which may contribute to cell damage.

The plant-based Ayurvedic diet contributes to balanced nutritional support, which is essential for stimulating the activity of immune system cells such as killer T-cells, which can destroy cancer cells before they develop into tumors. If you already have cancer, and are currently using conventional treatment, the Ayurvedic diet—along with massage, meditation, and other therapies—can be especially helpful in restoring balance, which can make a significant difference when your body is exhausted and you're frightened and anxious.

Another aspect of Ayurveda of interest to cancer survivors is the use of medicinal herbs, some of which are helpful for coping with the consequences of cancer. For example, if you're undergoing chemotherapy or radiation treatments, you may experience bone-wearying fatigue—understandably from the treatments, and perhaps due to sleep disturbances brought on by anxiety. Under such circumstances, an Ayurvedic practitioner might recommend the use of sedative herbs specific to your mind/body type that interacts with the same chemicals in the brain affected by conventional antianxiety drugs.

Ayurvedic practitioners also make use of ashwagandha, which reportedly enhances immunity and reduces stress; gotu kola, which improves sleep; ginkgo, which has powerful antioxidant effects; and ginger, which has been shown to reduce nausea. Unique combinations of herbs are associated with specific effects for balancing doshas and treating existing imbalances with symptomatic presentation. One should note that because herbal medicine plays such an important role in Ayurvedic medicine and the reliability of herbal resources can vary significantly, it is important to ascertain the source and quality of herbs being used for this purpose from your practitioner.

Dr. Carson recommends Ayurveda for her patients with cancer. She finds that they usually experience an improvement in energy levels soon after starting treatment. In addition, most of the techniques of Ayurveda can easily be incorporated into a self-care plan. "My recommendations vary, depending on what phase of treatment the individual is in," she says. "The techniques can be adapted for people in any stage of ease or dis-ease."

■ WHAT TO EXPECT ■

Ayurvedic treatment relies heavily on practitioner evaluation and recommendations, followed by self-care. When a patient first comes to the office, she or he is evaluated to determine individual mind/body type. This will in large part determine the recommended course of action.

The mind/body type is ascertained through observation, patient feedback, and a physical exam that includes pulse evaluation, examination of the tongue, urine, eyes, and nails, and palpation of organs.

Focus then shifts to rebalancing and reconnecting the patient to his or her inner source of vitality. The tools and practices used to achieve balance are specific to the individual's mind/body type and function within the framework of the individual's level of need, circumstance, and motivation.

A highly individualized treatment program may consist of a combination of some form of detoxification (known as Panchakarma treatments), such as herbs, herbal oil massages, or herbal steam saunas; palliation (balance created using herbs, diet, and fasting); neurorespiratory balance produced by breathing exercises; and meditative practices. Sound and light therapy are also prescribed in Ayurvedic practice. In other words, one uses all the senses to restore one's state of health and prevent illness.

Practitioners are well versed in nutritional counseling, because diet plays such a vital role in health, and specific foods are thought to have a positive or negative impact on particular doshas. Patients may also be advised about yoga, exercise, changes in daily habits, meditation, and breathing techniques, or they may be provided with herbal medicines for prevention, restoration, or for a specific condition, such as side effects from chemotherapy, for example.

Initial sessions with an Ayurvedic practitioner range from forty-five minutes to two hours. Patients may meet with a patient educator as well as the practitioner. Most programs include one or two follow-up sessions to evaluate progress, institute any changes to the treatment, and answer patient questions.

■ TRAINING ■

There are a multitude of training programs and Ayurvedic medical colleges for Ayurvedic physicians available throughout India, with varying requirements for qualifications and credentials. Training in the West is more limited. In the United States, there are several training programs in Ayurvedic medicine and Maharishi Ayur-Ved^{SM}* that range in quality and scope from instruction in diagnosis and treatment for medical doctors to programs that provide training to lay people which limits Ayurvedic practice to consultations only. Because of this disparity, it is important to investigate the qualifications and level of training of individual practitioners.

For instance, the Maharishi College of Vedic Medicine^{SM} currently offers a twelve-day training program to M.D.s, D.O.s, chiropractors, licensed naturopathic physicians, physician assistants, and nurse practitioners on the basic fundamentals of Vedic medicine and clinical training in diagnosis and the development of treatment plans. The Ayurvedic Institute provides a program for laypeople that includes training in herbology, yoga, and meditation, and a more in-depth, six-month Gurukula program for physicians. Another example is the California College of Ayurveda, which offers a two-year, 500-hour California state-approved clinical training program leading to certification as a clinical Ayurvedic specialist.

The National Institute of Ayurvedic Medicine (NIAM), in collaboration with the Institute of Indian Medicine and the University of Pune, is in the process of establish-

---

Ayurvedic medicine and Maharishi Ayur-Ved have both evolved from the traditional health practices of India, and both employ meditation as part of their treatment program. Maharishi Ayur-Ved, however, incorporates Transcendental Meditation®, a mantra-based meditation, as an integral part of treatment. It is considered by some to be an approach that differs from traditional Ayurveda.

ing the first India-approved certification program of study in Ayurvedic medicine in the United States. The three-year program will be taught by senior faculty of India's Ayurvedic colleges. Admission requires completion of at least two years of college and graduation from a formal program of training in a health care discipline.

States currently do not recognize Ayurveda as an independent health discipline. Efforts are under way in several states to recognize Ayurveda as a health profession and license it. Health insurance coverage for Ayurveda is available only under the health care practitioner's primary specialty.

■ TREATMENTS FROM TOP PRACTITIONERS ■

Kumuda Reddy, M.D., *is a physician practicing Ayurvedic medicine in Bethesda, Maryland. She has practiced a style of Ayurvedic medicine called Maharishi Vedic Medicine*^{SM} *since 1990.*

Treatment Goals

"Cancer is a very complicated disease," says Dr. Reddy. "We believe that cancer cells lose the memory of perfect cellular functioning that is innate in every cell in our bodies. When that memory of well-being is lost, a cancerous cell becomes dysfunctional and acts in whatever way it wants."

Maharishi Vedic Medicine is consciousness-based, Dr. Reddy explains. "It enlivens the body's inner intelligence to stimulate and enhance internal self-repair mechanisms, so healing can occur naturally from within. It essentially connects with and stimulates healing from the deepest levels of consciousness."

With Maharishi Vedic Medicine, the biological inner intelligence can be restored, Dr. Reddy explains. "There are so many aspects that need to be addressed with the cancer patient: ensuring overall well-being, increasing the quality of life, improving digestion and sleep, reducing anxiety and depression, and supporting the ability to carry on with normal activities and have peace of mind," she says.

The Ayurvedic approach of Maharishi Vedic Medicine balances, heals, and rejuvenates the mind, body, and emotions. Dr. Reddy believes it can help cancer patients to know they are much more than their cancer and evolve beyond whatever limitations they have.

Treatment Session

At the initial session, the patient is asked to complete history forms, which emphasize lifestyle, emotional make-up, life stresses, digestion, elimination, and sleep. After

MY APPROACH

Catherine K. Carson, D.C., C.Ad., a certified Ayurvedic physician and doctor of chiropractic in Fairfax, Virginia, has been in practice for more than fifteen years.

"My goal is always to give people the information and tools that they need to get to the most perfect state of health at any given time. In Ayurveda, the basic constitution of the individual remains unaltered during his or her lifetime. The combination of elements that governs the continuous physiopathology in the body alters in response to changes in the environment. The goal of Ayurveda is to provide the tools one can use to maintain one's state of health and well-being in the face of these environmental changes.

"Ayurvedic medicine is most useful to cancer patients in that it provides easy access to another realm of alternative approaches and easy, 'do-it-yourself' methods of health care, which is healing in and of itself.

"During my initial consultation, there's a brief physical exam, which includes a pulse and blood pressure check as well as a determination of the individual mind/body type, which is essential in Ayurvedic medicine.

"Based on the findings of the physical exam and an extensive health history, I develop a set of recommendations for diet, sleep, exercise, and

Dr. Reddy reviews the patient's history, she performs a pulse diagnosis, and may collect blood samples for additional analysis. Dr. Reddy then discusses her findings and makes recommendations to the patient for various Maharishi Ayur-Veda modalities.

According to Dr. Reddy, the Transcendental Meditation® technique facilitates the enlivenment of consciousness and stimulates healing on a deeper level. In addition, dietary changes are suggested to balance the body's physiology. Balanced herbal formulations are often recommended to cleanse, nourish, and rejuvenate. Other treatments used by Dr. Reddy include Maharishi Vedic Vibration Technology℠ and Maharishi Rejuvenation℠ treatments.

A total of forty-five to sixty minutes are spent in con-

---

daily activity. In the broadest sense, the goal is to help people achieve a more positive state of mental-physical well-being. The treatment can also be fine-tuned to reduce fatigue, nausea, or other side effects from conventional cancer treatments.

"I really look at each individual to see what his or her needs are. I teach Ayurvedic methods in ways that are easy to administer, which is why a lot of my clients are able to stay committed to self-care.

"Because the underlying principles of Ayurveda are so complex, the consultations are much longer than they would be with a conventional physician. Those with cancer may need more extensive supervision and usually come to the office monthly.

"I believe that Ayurvedic treatment is a productive adjunct to conventional cancer care, and I do make adjustments depending on what's happening with the patient's treatment. For example, I don't recommend that people use strong antioxidant nutrients on the days when chemotherapy is being administered. I also discourage deep tissue or lymphatic massage for those dealing with lymphatic cancers. Apart from this, massage, hot oil treatments, and most dietary measures are very compatible with conventional treatments."

sultation with Dr. Reddy, followed by a meeting with the center's patient educator. Here, further explanation is given on the diagnosis and recommended treatments, and any additional questions are answered. Usually the entire intake session is scheduled for two and a half hours. A second visit is scheduled in three to four weeks, when the patient is re-evaluated.

Benefits to Cancer Patients

Dr. Reddy believes that the treatments support the cancer patient by improving the body's natural ability to heal. Digestion and metabolism are strengthened, side effects from conventional treatments are lessened, vitality is increased, and overall quality of life is improved.

Compatibility with Conventional Treatment

"As a medical doctor and Ayurvedic physician, I am not opposed to conventional cancer treatment," says Dr. Reddy. "But I believe that when conventional treatment is used, Maharishi Ayur-Veda treatments should be there as well. The Maharishi Vedic Medicine approach to health brings you back to who you are, to that intimate connection to the deeper levels of our being."

FOR FURTHER INFORMATION

Contact the organizations listed below for further information on training, referrals, Ayurvedic medicine, and Maharishi Ayur-Ved products and services.

The Maharishi College of Vedic Medicine
2721 Arizona Street, NE
Albuquerque, NM 87110
(505) 830-0415
www.mcvm-nm.org

The Ayurvedic Institute
11311 Menaul NE
Albuquerque, NM 87112
(505) 291-9698
www.ayurveda.com

The California College of Ayurveda
1117A East Main Street
Grass Valley, CA 95945
(530) 274-9100
www.ayurvedacollege.com

National Institute of Ayurvedic Medicine
584 Milltown Road
Brewster, NY 10509
(845) 278-8700
www.niam.com

Deepak Chopra, M.D., has been influential in introducing Ayurvedic medicine to this country through his writings and other work. The Chopra Center at La Costa Resort and Spa offers wellness retreats, treatments, and instruction in Ayurveda and other complementary therapies. You might wish to visit his web site at www.chopra.com for more information.

The Chopra Center at La Costa Resort and Spa
2013 Costa del Mar Road
Carlsbad, CA 92009
(888) 424-6772

Maharishi Ayur-Ved Products International, Inc. (MAPI), supplier of Ayurvedic formulas, provides a listing of Maharishi Ayur-Ved physicians by state. The list can be obtained by calling (800) 345-8332. Their web site is www.mapi.com.

BOOKS RECOMMENDED BY HEALERS

The Ayurvedic Cookbook. Amadea Morningstar and Urmila Desai (Santa Fe, New Mexico: Lotus Press, 1990).

Ayurveda: The Science of Self-Healing: A Practical Guide. **Vasant Lad (Santa Fe, New Mexico: Lotus Press, 1984).**

Forever Healthy: Introduction to Maharishi Ayur-Veda Health Care: Preventing and Treating Disease Through Timeless Natural Medicine. **Kumuda Reddy and Stan Kendz (Rochester, New York: Samhita Enterprises, Inc., 1997).**

Perfect Health: The Complete Mind/Body Guide. **Deepak Chopra (New York: Harmony Books, 1991).**

Prakruti: Your Ayurvedic Constitution. **Robert E. Svoboda (Albuquerque, New Mexico: GEOCO, 1988).**

A wide variety of systems and techniques can be categorized as bodywork. What they have in common is the use of touch as a therapeutic tool to heal the body, calm the mind, and soothe the spirit.

Many cancer patients turn to one or more of the various types of bodywork at any point during their treatment or recovery. There are so many options to choose from that nearly everyone can find a system that feels comfortable and right. Bodywork is commonly used to control stress, but many of the different forms also affect the body's ability to cope with cancer or other illnesses—by supporting proper immune system functioning, aiding in flexibility and movement, reducing pain, and nurturing the spirit.

Bodywork therapies encompass structural techniques, movement, massage, and energy balancing. Their boundaries can seem quite fluid because many bodywork practitioners combine different methods. In addition, some techniques are known both as "bodywork" and as "energetic healing" or "energy medicine." In this section, I focus on techniques that are more manual in their delivery than the modalities described in a later section on Energy Healing.

BODYWORK AND HEALING

Although some bodywork therapies are more contemporary than others, the use of touch in a therapeutic role has been popular in many cultures for centuries. It has been studied widely and proven effective in managing pain; improving body structure, motion, and function; assisting in detoxification; and assisting in healing both acute and chronic musculoskeletal conditions. Some forms of bodywork promote better circulation and reduce swelling, inflammation, and scar tissue adhesions.

Bodywork can lead clients to greater self-awareness and increase vitality and well-being. It also has powerful emotional effects, which can be of particular importance to cancer patients. Different forms of bodywork can reduce stress, relieve fatigue (emotional or physical) caused by illness or cancer treatments, help release emotions, and generally produce uplifting or restorative effects.

Just as the boundaries of bodywork remain fluid, so, I believe, should your selection of techniques. The variety of approaches and outcomes each therapy offers makes it important to try different treatments to find what is most effective for your needs and circumstances. As your body heals, you may also find that a different technique or therapy is a better match for you than your current mode of treatment.

Having said that, I would caution you as a cancer patient to begin any bodywork only under the advice and consent of your physician. Certain conditions (such as inflammation, circulatory problems, or acute infection) may be contraindicated for some bodywork. Keep your complementary practitioner (or practitioners) well informed of your physical situation and any constraints.

In the following pages I'll describe a variety of bodywork therapies. This is not a comprehensive guide to all available bodywork systems. There are many wonderful resources available for further research, some of which I have listed here. I would encourage you to further investigate therapies that interest you.

ALEXANDER TECHNIQUE

The Alexander Technique, which focuses mainly on balance, is based on the premise that there is an ideal alignment of the head, neck, and spine that promotes and supports proper movement, balance, posture, and overall physical and emotional functioning. The techniques developed by F. M. Alexander approximately one hundred years ago help to restore a person's natural alignment, resulting in better distribution of musculoskeletal support, movement, and response.

These techniques are not considered healing treatments, but rather skills taught to clients so that old postural, movement, and reacting habits can be corrected and body awareness can be improved.

Yet the Alexander Technique can often be helpful to cancer patients. Once people learn the techniques, they often find that they feel better emotionally as well as physically. Some of the lessons make it easier for clients to overcome weakness or balance problems, let go of debilitating fears, and even breathe more naturally and with less effort.

The Alexander Technique is usually taught over a course of thirty individual lessons. Basic movements are guided through the teacher's touch and verbal support. The focus of the lessons is on identifying and correcting any dysfunction in movement or posture, and on redirecting responses to external stimuli, or stressors.

■ HOW IT HELPS ■

The Alexander Technique has been used to treat many conditions, ranging from muscle spasms, skeletal strain, and nerve pain to chronic pain associated with movement, chronic fatigue, and postsurgical weakness. It has also been used successfully as a stress management technique.

"Most patients come in for physical pain," says Lynn Brice Rosen, a certified Alexander Technique instructor in Washington, D.C. "With the Alexander Technique, people are better able to balance in the face of stress," she says. "It's a very pragmatic technique that opens many layers of support and discovery."

Coping with pain will always be a challenge for cancer patients. Apart from the discomfort of the illness itself, the current treatments put tremendous stress on the body. Women who have had surgery for breast cancer, for example, may find that their neck and shoulders hurt for months afterward. Often, surgery can change—usually temporarily, but sometimes for years—the body's natural pattern of movements. This can lead to increased muscle strain as the body attempts to compensate for the loss of balance and natural strength.

The Alexander Technique addresses balance problems, such as those caused by neuropathy, prosthesis imbalance, weakness, or surgery, and increases range of motion, strength, and flexibility. With the Alexander Technique, clients learn how to move and even sit and stand in ways that put the least strain on the body. Cancer patients who practice the techniques also can discover ways to modulate their response to pain, which can reduce its intensity and make it easier to control.

■ WHAT TO EXPECT ■

Sessions can last from thirty to sixty minutes; the time depends on how quickly clients make progress. Most people who study the Alexander Technique will do so in a series of sessions ranging from twenty to forty lessons. Instructors often advise clients that frequent repetition makes it easier to learn the different techniques.

Because the Alexander Technique teaches movement and posture skills, clients are advised to wear comfortable clothing. The instructor will begin by observing the client's posture and movement patterns, to get a sense of what may need correcting. Rather than merely describing proper alignment, the instructor touches the neck, shoulders, back, and other parts of the body, using gentle pressure to show what's required.

As sessions progress and clients discover how to move their bodies in a more harmonious fashion, they often experience a release of muscular tension, as well as a reduction in pain and discomfort.

■ TRAINING ■

Certified Alexander Technique teachers receive 1,600 hours of training over a minimum of three years (part-time) in a school certified by the American Society for the Alexander Technique (AmSAT). Application for certification is reviewed by AmSAT upon completion of training. There are currently eighteen certified AmSAT training programs in the United States. (Other training programs exist that are not certified by AmSAT.) States do not regulate the profession; very few health insurance programs provide coverage.

■ TREATMENTS FROM TOP PRACTITIONERS ■

Lynn Brice Rosen *is a certified Alexander Technique instructor at the Body College in Washington, D.C. She has worked with many cancer survivors over the years.*

Treatment Goals

"I give my clients a means by which they can have more choices over their responses to whatever is troubling them: emotional pain, anxiety, fear, anticipation, physical pain—anything they are facing," Rosen says. "I offer them the tools that allow them, at a minimum, to be in parallel with their situation, so that the powerful, dark feelings don't overwhelm them."

People who learn the Alexander Technique are able to think more clearly, Rosen adds. They may find they have more clarity about their purpose and goals, even when they're in the midst of dealing with cancer.

"People who have faced a life-threatening illness have already begun to prioritize their lives. But as they learn this method of energy efficiency, their lists of "musts" and "shoulds" begin to change. Not only do they learn more about the mechanics of their body, they learn to find balance in the world."

Treatment Session

Rosen's initial work with clients involves balancing the head on the spine to conserve energy and achieve proper balance. Typical sessions include bodywork on the table (using books to support the head), and upright work involving daily activities, such as walking, bending, reaching, standing, and sitting. The goal is to improve the basic body mechanics, thereby bringing the person into better harmony. Ms. Rosen uses a very light touch, stimulating the reflexes to create more space and ease.

Each session lasts forty-five minutes. After ten sessions, Rosen recommends that clients assess how well they've been able to integrate the treatments into their lives.

It's not uncommon for some people to experience disorientation at first, she says. "They sometimes feel lighter, higher, smoother, more relaxed, softer, and more steady. Sometimes it takes feeling off balance to experience new balance," she says. Initially, some people may feel stiff or sore after the sessions, but most people have very positive responses.

Benefits to Cancer Patients

The Alexander Technique can benefit cancer patients in a variety of ways. Those who have had mastectomies, need prosthetics, or suffer from neuropathy or post-treatment weakness can learn to restore—or improve—their sense of balance and physical control. "I help them discover ways to manage pain and improve the efficiency of their basic movement skills, such as getting in and out of the bath, carrying groceries, or simply walking or sitting," says Rosen.

If you're recovering from surgery, the Alexander Technique can be a powerful and wonderful tool, Rosen says. Some patients report that they require less pain medication after learning the techniques.

Compatibility with Conventional Treatment
Ms. Rosen sees no adverse effects from combining the Alexander Technique with conventional cancer treatments. She encourages her patients to discuss the lessons with their oncologists or physicians, and she's happy to work closely with physicians to monitor patient progress.

FOR FURTHER INFORMATION
Contact the American Society for the Alexander Technique (AmSAT) at (800) 473-0620, or www.alexandertech.com for a nationwide list of over four hundred certified Alexander Technique teachers.
American Society for the Alexander Technique
P.O. Box 60008, Suite 10
Florence, Massachusetts 01062

BOOKS RECOMMENDED BY HEALERS
Back Trouble: A New Approach to Prevention and Recovery. **Deborah Caplan** (Gainesville, Florida: Triad Publishing Company, 1987).

How to Learn the Alexander Technique: A Manual for Students. **Barbara Conable and William Conable** (Columbus, Ohio: Andover Road Press, 1992).

A New Approach to the Alexander Technique: Moving Toward a More Balanced Expression of the Whole Self. **Glen Park** (Freedom, California: Crossing Press, 1998).

CRANIOSACRAL THERAPY

This form of bodywork was inspired by osteopathic medicine, but its focus is solely on the craniosacral system, which includes the cerebrospinal fluid and head, spine, and pelvic bones. Through craniosacral therapy, certain natural rhythms of the central nervous system and body are monitored and utilized to improve body function. Cancer patients may find the treatment useful in that it may relieve some of the emotional and physical dysfunctions that accompany cancer, including stress, muscle stiffness, or muscle and joint pain.

■ HOW IT HELPS ■

Craniosacral therapy is used to treat nervous system dysfunctions and structural misalignment, as well as muscle tension and injuries. For those with cancer, one of its main benefits is to help cope with stress, which can contribute to persistent muscle pain or fatigue. Stress also weakens immunity, which reduces the body's ability to combat foreign cells in the body, including cancer cells.

As with other forms of hands-on therapy, craniosacral therapy, by gently manipulating the anatomy of the head, spine, and pelvis, dilates blood vessels and increases the flow of blood and lymphatic fluid, which contributes to healing and recovery. The supply of oxygen to the tissues increases, and muscles that may have been weakened as a result of cancer or cancer treatments can be stimulated. The gentle touch that's used in craniosacral therapy can also relieve some common physical symptoms cancer patients experience, such as headaches, insomnia, or back pain.

When working with cancer patients, a primary goal is to help them resolve psychological/emotional stress and trauma, says Ronald Murray, N.D., P.T., a naturopathic physician, physical therapist, and craniosacral practitioner in Silver Spring, Maryland.

"If you have a chronic, life-threatening illness, and you feel you have some unresolved psychological issues—especially if you have been through psychotherapy already without complete resolution of your issues—then this treatment is for you," he says. "A lot of people I see respond to this work when no other treatment has helped them." Although it won't affect the progress of the disease, craniosacral therapy can significantly boost feelings of well-being and improve the quality of life.

■ WHAT TO EXPECT ■

The practitioner employs a very light touch to assess the natural, rhythmic movement of the craniosacral system. Through very gentle adjustment, the flow of cerebrospinal fluid is increased and any blocks to that flow are removed. Improved flow of cerebrospinal fluid is believed to help balance the central nervous system (CNS) and support proper functioning of the entire body. Over time, the musculoskeletal system becomes more relaxed, and clients may feel an increase in energy.

■ TRAINING ■

Craniosacral therapy is practiced by massage therapists and other professional bodyworkers, osteopaths, chiropractors, physical therapists, and other health care professionals trained in the technique. Training in craniosacral therapy is offered as continuing education to health care practitioners licensed or certified under their major specialty area, through craniosacral training and certification programs. Some massage schools offer training in craniosacral therapy as part of their ancillary curriculum.

The Upledger Institute, Inc.® in Florida is a well-known provider of several complementary modality training programs including CranioSacral™ Therapy, and has established the American CranioSacral™ Therapy Association.

Training in craniosacral therapy differs from instruction in cranial osteopathy. Cranial osteopathy is offered as part of the curriculum in osteopathic medical schools. In addition, allopathic and osteopathic physicians and dentists can be trained in this approach through continuing medical educational studies. It is considered a medical procedure.

As with any modality you are researching, it is wise to investigate the training and experience of your practitioners.

State regulation and health insurance coverage vary by state and the caregiver's primary health care specialty (for example, physical therapy, massage therapy, etc.).

■ **TREATMENTS FROM TOP PRACTITIONERS** ■
Ronald Murray, N.D., P.T., *is a naturopathic physician, physical therapist, and practitioner of craniosacral therapy at the Asclepion Center for Body Mind Therapy in Silver Spring, Maryland.*

Treatment Goals

Dr. Murray believes that with every illness, there may be an emotional or psychological basis, as well as a physical expression. "Even though psychological or emotional factors may not be the cause of the illness, they can be factors that prevent the person from moving forward in his or her healing process," he says.

"With cancer patients, I try to look at what the internal environment is like—where there are restrictions to energy flow. My goal is to give the person an opportunity to resolve any deeply held traumas that may be inhibiting healing. The work I do interrupts or alters deeply ingrained energy patterns, which hopefully will interrupt or alter the course or the energy pattern of the cancer."

Treatment Session

Dr. Murray's initial assessment begins as soon as a client enters his office. "How they walk, sit, and carry themselves begins to tell me what's going on," he notes.

Dr. Murray first obtains a health history, and gives the client literature that describes the different therapies he may be using. The client removes his or her shoes and lies down on a massage table. There might be background music to help the patient relax, as Dr. Murray believes it's important for clients to be in an emotional place where they can receive the work.

"I place my hands on different parts of the body: when I 'listen' with my hands, the body directs me to what the internal needs are at that particular time," he says. "All tissue has an inherent movement. When I gently touch the body, I can feel an attraction to tissue that isn't moving—and then I determine if the restriction is psycho-emotional or mechanical. For me, the energies are very different between the two."

Dr. Murray explains that in using craniosacral therapy and other techniques, he "engages" the energy until it's ready to unbind itself. As blocks are removed or dispersed, the body and spirit move a bit closer to the natural state of balance, alignment, and optimal healing capacity.

The sessions usually last for sixty minutes, and they're scheduled weekly. Significant changes are usually observed within four to six sessions. During the treatments, clients most often report feelings of warmth or tingling. It's not uncommon for the treatments to stir up old memories, feelings, tears, and vivid dreams.

But Dr. Murray stresses that craniosacral therapy is unique to each patient: everyone's response to the treatments will be highly individualized.

Benefits to Cancer Patients

Dr. Murray notes that in addition to relieving psychological/emotional stress and trauma, craniosacral therapy improves the body's physiology, lessens pain, improves energy and blood flow, and increases overall well-being.

Compatibility with Conventional Treatment

Dr. Murray sees no conflict between his therapy and cancer treatment. At his clinic he works with physicians and is willing to coordinate care with clients' oncologists if they so choose.

FOR FURTHER INFORMATION

The Upledger Institute publishes a directory of the International Association of Healthcare Practitioners (IAHP), which lists over forty thousand Upledger alumni by their credentials and location. Copies can be purchased by calling (800) 311-9204, or by accessing their web site, www.iahp.com. State listings of IAHP members can be retrieved on the web site. (Note that graduates of other craniosacral certification programs are not included in this listing, and may be accessed through schools of bodywork in your area.)

The Cranial Academy, an organization associated with the American Academy of Osteopathy, promotes and teaches cranial osteopathy. For more information on cranial osteopathy or to obtain a referral for a practitioner of cranial osteopathy (physicians and dentists only), contact the Cranial Academy at (317) 594-0411, or visit their web site, www.cranialacademy.org.

American CranioSacral Therapy Association
11211 Prosperity Farms Road, Suite D-325
Palm Beach Gardens, FL 33410-3487
(800) 233-5880

The Cranial Academy
8202 Clearvista Parkway, Suite 9-D
Indianapolis, IN 46256
(317) 594-0411

BOOKS RECOMMENDED BY HEALERS
Your Inner Physician and You: CranioSacral Therapy and SomatoEmotional Release®.
John E. Upledger (Berkeley, California: North Atlantic Books, 1997).

MASSAGE

This well-known treatment has enjoyed thousands of years of use in many cultures, assisting in stress reduction, muscle relaxation, restoration, and rejuvenation on an energetic as well as a physical level.

Therapeutic massage employs specific physical techniques to manipulate muscles and soft tissues. The goal of massage is the prevention and reduction of muscle tension which, unabated, can lead to muscle fatigue and nerve compression, and can contribute to chronic stress patterns and pain elsewhere in the body.

■ HOW IT HELPS ■

Massage has been reported to be helpful in treating conditions ranging from headaches, backaches, and muscle spasms to high blood pressure and depression. Many cancer patients turn to massage because it helps relax the nervous system, reduces stress, and increases the capacity for a clearer, calmer mind. Touch has been found to be extremely useful in grief and loss work as well. Massage nourishes both mind and body; the physical relaxation one experiences during massage can release emotions, lower anxiety, soothe tension, and give an emotional lift.

On a purely physical level, massage improves circulation, which helps the natural healing process after illness.

Massage can reduce swelling and improve breathing, posture, and motion. It appears to stimulate the body's ability to combat pain, which can be helpful for controlling discomfort caused by cancer—from both the disease itself and the various treatments that are used.

For cancer patients, the value of massage and other touch treatments has been well documented. For instance, a study published in the journal *Cancer Nursing* found that hospitalized cancer patients who were given a thirty-minute therapeutic massage on two consecutive evenings had a 60 percent reduction in pain levels, and a 24 percent reduction in anxiety.[10] A pilot study of 29 cancer patients conducted by the University of Washington in 2000 showed a 42 percent reduction in pain in the group receiving four twice-weekly massages, compared with a 25 percent pain reduction in the control group.[11]

Fear and anxiety are nearly universal among cancer patients, and the negative effects of these emotions range from a sense of helplessness to depressed immunity—which could affect the body's ability to deal with cancer or other illnesses. When people are frightened or anxious, the body releases stress hormones. Initially, these hormones increase levels of white blood cells as part of the body's defensive posture. When stress hormones remain high, however, white blood cell numbers are reduced, weakening the body's ability to protect itself from threats.

"I try to help my clients see that their body is not the enemy," says Ricey Clapp, a massage practitioner and physician assistant in Silver Spring, Maryland. "Even with cancer, you are still able to heal and change. Healing—both emotional and physical—is helped so much when one can see how restoring health to one area impacts the rest of the body."

In a study at Kessler Medical Rehabilitation and Education Corporation in West Orange, New Jersey, researchers looked at the link between massage and immune function.[12] They found that 56 percent of those who received massage had substantial increases in immune function. Specifically, they had increased numbers of white blood cells as well as an increase in natural killer cell activity. Researchers at the University of Miami also found increases in natural killer cells in women with breast cancer after they received massages.[13]

Massage may be particularly beneficial for cancer patients following surgery. After surgery, fluids may accumulate in the lymphatic system, causing discomfort or restricted movement. Massage can be effective in stimulating the body's waste-removal systems to work more efficiently, removing toxins and excessive fluids from the body.

The most common reason people employ massage is because it's relaxing. For those with cancer or other illnesses, spending an hour on the massage table provides a welcome relief from stress and anxiety. The beneficial effects of massage can extend beyond relaxation, and persist even after the sessions are completed.

■ WHAT TO EXPECT ■

Massage is an umbrella term that includes more than a hundred different techniques—everything from deep tissue and Swedish massage to the more gentle techniques employed in craniosacral treatments and specialized techniques such as manual lymph drainage used for lymphedema, a condition that is often a side effect of cancer treatment.

When clients arrive at the office, they're usually ushered into a quiet, dimly lit room. Massage is usually performed on a massage table, with the client unclothed (although some massage therapists will work with the client fully clothed). Modesty is preserved during treatments because most of the body remains covered by a sheet; portions of the sheet will be moved aside to expose small areas of skin, then re-covered when the therapist moves to a different area.

The therapist may begin by asking if there are any sore or tense areas that need particular attention. During the session, the therapist will apply a small amount of oil to his or her hands, and begin the massage. The client will be asked if the massage strokes are too light or too vigorous. Once the approach has been refined, the therapist will massage the entire body, usually for sixty to ninety minutes.

■ TRAINING ■

There are approximately one thousand massage training schools in this country, both American Massage Therapy Association (AMTA) and non-AMTA member schools. AMTA-approved training programs require five hundred training hours; some states require one thousand hours.

The National Certification Board for Therapeutic Massage and Bodywork (NCBTMB) is a voluntary national credentialing program that assures the basic competency of practitioners of various forms of therapeutic massage and bodywork. Certification is dependent upon certain eligibility requirements and demonstration of competency. Over forty thousand therapists of various bodywork modalities (therapeutic massage in particular) are currently certified through the NCBTMB. Note that this certification is not specific to nor sought by practitioners of all bodywork modalities.

The massage therapy profession is currently in a period of significant growth, change, and expansion. At this writing, twenty-nine states and the District of Columbia have passed some form of legislation regulating the massage profession with either licensure, certification, or registration. Health insurance coverage for massage therapy may be available through some companies in states that license massage therapy.

■ TREATMENTS OF TOP PRACTITIONERS ■

Mary Beebe and Sandy Truxell, *both certified massage therapists, offer massage, therapeutic healing touch, and reiki to patients in Cotuit, Massachusetts (Beebe) and Reston, Virginia (Truxell). They offer a wide range of bodywork techniques to their clients.*

Treatment Goals

Beebe and Truxell agree that "the major goal for cancer patients in seeking massage is stress reduction, because as soon as you reduce stress, it can alleviate other problems. If you've been through multiple medical procedures and touched in ways that are uncomfortable, then being touched in a comfortable way is vastly important to healing. It's very gratifying to send people who are stressed out from our offices in a more relaxed state."

Truxell emphasizes that in their practice, "we aren't working *on* a client; rather, it is an exchange. We work with each other—the client and the practitioner—so that the hour is spent in a very safe, protected space in which the client can let go. The skin is our connection to the outside world: when we touch another, we contact the individual's body, mind, and spirit with our own. It's a profoundly spiritual experience to be allowed to work so intimately with another individual."

Treatment Session

Both Beebe and Truxell offer one-hour sessions, but vary slightly in their approach. Beebe spends ten minutes initially with her clients, obtaining a brief health history and discussing current issues. Then the patient lies down, unclothed, on a massage table. Using music and oils, Beebe begins her massage at the head, working down the front of the body and then the back. Beebe also offers healing touch and gentle myofascial release work for chronic pain, if the client requests.

Beebe recommends Swedish massage weekly, particularly during chemotherapy or radiation. "I encourage my cancer clients to make a commitment to nurture themselves, whether it is once a week or twice a month, as it is so important to healing," she says.

Truxell's bodywork practice includes therapeutic touch and reiki along with her massage treatments. She begins her intake session by taking a detailed medical history. "I tailor each treatment session, and am particularly respectful of any past traumas and particular physical needs," she says. Truxell refrains from using scented oils because of clients' allergies and sensitivities. Clients may be clothed or undressed during treatments.

Benefits to Cancer Patients

Both Beebe and Truxell believe that massage stimulates the immune system, decreases depression and feelings of hope-

---

MY APPROACH

Ricey Clapp is a massage practitioner and licensed physician assistant in Silver Spring, Maryland. She also incorporates aromatherapy into her practice.

"My goal is to help cancer patients reclaim and restore structural integrity to their bodies. By working with the body's systems—emphasizing the connective tissue system—I try to integrate the body to promote better function overall.

"For cancer patients, my treatments can promote increased energy and more symmetrical motion, as well as a greater ability to meet physical activity challenges. People often experience an increased sense of well-being as they reclaim their bodies' function without fear of pain or injury.

"My sessions focus on structural bodywork and are highly individualized. For instance, biomechanical work sometimes requires a lot of movelessness, reduces stress, and improves the body overall. They report that massage affects the body's normal relaxation response, and can bring about physical and emotional release, often easing pain and helping to create a more positive outlook as one heals. Beebe observes that "muscles feel better, the body feels better; some people find it to be a great emotional release, and it appears to help with treatment side effects as well." Truxell has found that "massage helps relieve physical pain, improve sleep, and is a wonderful way to exchange energy." Both agree that, overall, "people just feel better after massage."

Compatibility with Conventional Treatment

Both practitioners see no incompatibility with massage and conventional cancer treatment, unless the cancer is systemic. In this case, gentle healing work, such as therapeutic touch or healing touch (as opposed to more rigorous massage), can still be offered if the client is comfortable with that approach. Truxell and Beebe require all

---

ment on the client's part, so a light massage might be appropriate. Many sessions are devoted to aromatherapy massage. This involves applying an individualized blend of essential oils to the body—it's a wonderfully relaxing and nurturing treatment, very different in intent and effect from the popular Swedish massage, which tends to knead the muscles more deeply and may be more stimulating. I have found that aromatherapy lifts cancer patients' spirits and reduces stress. My patients report feeling especially peaceful and nurtured following an aromatherapy massage.

"The bodywork I perform is gentle. Most clients report little discomfort, although if they're new to structural bodywork, they may initially experience some tenderness. Some discomfort may be positive because it demonstrates that people are responding to the treatment. Cancer patients deserve special sensitivity given their experience."

clients to disclose current conditions and medications, noting that they prefer to coordinate care with their clients' physicians when dealing with cancer.

FOR FURTHER INFORMATION

The American Massage Therapy Association (AMTA) is the largest international organization for massage therapists. Contact the AMTA at (888) 843-2682 (THE-AMTA). Find a Massage Therapist℠ is a national locator service for AMTA professional members who agree to be listed and meet specific requirements. The locator service can be accessed through their web site, www.amtamassage.org .

American Massage Therapy Association
820 Davis Street, Suite 100
Evanston, IL 60201-4444
(847) 864-0123

NCBTMB certification requirements and a list of NCBTMB certified practitioners for your area can also be obtained through the NCBTMB at (800) 296-0664, or www.ncbtmb.com .

National Certification Board for Therapeutic Massage and Bodywork
8201 Greensboro Drive, Suite 300
McLean, VA 22102
(703) 610-9015

BOOKS RECOMMENDED BY HEALERS

The Book of Massage: The Complete Step-by-Step Guide to Eastern and Western Techniques. Lucinda Lidell (New York: Simon and Schuster, 1984).

The Complete Body Massage: A Hands-On Manual. Fiona Harrold (New York: Sterling Publishing Company, 1992).

Massage Made Easy. Mario-Paul Cassar (Allentown, Pennsylvania: People's Medical Society, 1995).

POLARITY THERAPY

Polarity therapy reflects the expertise and holistic beliefs of its originator, Dr. Randolph Stone, who practiced chiropractic, naturopathy, and osteopathy. Dr. Stone experienced the body as an electromagnetic system whose subtle energy currents may become out of balance in their polarity function of attraction and repulsion, expansion and contraction. Polarity therapy is based on a five-element system of life energy: ether, air, fire, water, and earth. Each element is believed to express varying frequencies of energy and embodies structures and processes in the body, such as the nervous system (air), and muscles and digestive organs (fire), with the ether element creating the space for movement and change.

As in other modalities, polarity therapy operates on the premise that illness stems from imbalanced or blocked energy (whether physical, emotional, or mental). Practitioners use a combination of therapeutic bodywork techniques, including gentle rocking, stretching, and pressure-sensitive touch. Practitioners also promote proper energy flow and balance through verbal guidance, counseling in cleansing and health-building diets, and teaching gentle stretching and breathing exercises, which encourage the client's participation in the healing process. The different techniques used in polarity therapy can relieve tension and make it easier for patients with cancer to tolerate standard medical treatments.

■ HOW IT HELPS ■

Polarity therapy aims to release blocked energy flow and balance the client's life energy. It therefore can result in emotional and physical release. According to Elaine Callinan, a registered polarity practitioner in Silver Spring, Maryland, bimanual (two-hand) contact facilitates the freeing-up of blocked energy into its natural direction of ease and movement. This enhanced circulation of energy, blood, oxygen, and lymphatic fluid cleanses and oxygenates muscle and organ tissues, soothes the nervous system, and relieves muscle pain and stiffness. Those that have used polarity therapy have also reported an increase in overall energy, flexibility, and clarity, along with a greater awareness of self and one's energetic patterns, enhanced well-being, and improved quality of life.

"Because cancer runs so deep, helping patients to access deeper levels of their being is essential to healing," says Callinan. "Patients must perceive themselves as something more than the medical model. By learning about the body's patterns from a holistic point of view, one can begin to feel the balance that is available, access resources in a more healthy fashion, and relate to the body as friend, guide, and teacher."

■ WHAT TO EXPECT ■

A typical polarity therapy session lasts sixty to ninety minutes. The practitioner may take a health history in the initial session, observing the client's behavior, posture, and movement patterns. The client, wearing comfortable, loose-fitting clothing, then moves to a massage table, where the practitioner may palpate, or touch, different parts of the body in order to assess energy movement. (Some polarity practitioners who are trained in massage may prefer less clothing in order to facilitate the application of massage techniques.)

Polarity therapy involves extensive hands-on work. A bimanual contact is utilized, with three types of touch: the very light, soothing satvic touch; gentle rocking (rajas), to stimulate energy flow; and deep contact to release contracted tissues in areas of extreme muscular tension (tamas). A polarity session also may include learning simple self-help movements and exercises, and dietary or life counseling, should the client demonstrate a lack of balance in these areas. Clients report that they feel changes in their energy patterns during and after treatments. They often leave the sessions with relief from pain and feeling deeply relaxed, invigorated, and peaceful.

■ TRAINING ■

The American Polarity Therapy Association (APTA), which accredits professional training for polarity therapists, recognizes two levels of certified training within the profession: associate polarity practitioner (APP), which currently requires 155 hours of training; and the more advanced registered polarity practitioner (RPP), which currently requires 650 hours of training and membership in APTA. There are approximately fifty approved RPP programs in the United States. Like massage, polarity therapy is in a period of rapid growth, change, and expansion; training and standards for practice are under continuous review and change.

Although polarity therapy is distinct from massage therapy, it is included under massage legislation in a few states. Health insurance coverage may be available in states that license massage therapy.

■ TREATMENTS FROM TOP PRACTITIONERS ■

Elaine Callinan *is a registered polarity practitioner in Silver Spring, Maryland. She has been in practice since 1990, and her work includes advanced massage and bodywork.*

Treatment Goals

Callinan believes that the body is a roadmap to the self and, as such, it reflects the whole being. "I work with the person as a hologram, through the medium of the body," Callinan says. "All aspects of a person—mind, emotions, and spirit—can be accessed through any body part or system. I work within a conceptual framework of structural-energy interface, so I work on several levels: muscular, connective tissue, nervous system, and energy movement. I try to introduce my clients to the processes of their body, to facilitate their becoming their own healers, and to build a relationship with the body as friend and teacher in a very practical way."

Treatment Session

Callinan allows ninety minutes for each session. The first twenty minutes is usually given to dialogue, which allows clients to establish a connection with her and express their needs and wishes. The initial intake information forms the basis for discussion of health issues.

The treatments are given on a massage table. Callinan can work with a client clothed, but prefers her clients to be unclothed; she believes that touch is important to healing. She never begins work on an area of the body that has been traumatized; rather, she nourishes any traumatized areas by working on related parts of the body, to relax and support the nervous system.

During treatments, Callinan uses her hands to ground the client, remove energy blocks to promote better circulation, release chronic holding patterns, and help people access a deeper level of healing.

Side effects from polarity treatments depend on a client's experience with body work, as well as his or her general state of health. The normal flow of body systems is disrupted as toxins are being moved and energy released. This can result in stiffness, emotional irritability, or discomfort for up to a day following treatment. She advises clients to drink lots of water and take a warm bath following treatment to alleviate any discomfort.

As clients have additional sessions, the body gets

accustomed to the treatments. She encourages people to discuss what they're feeling during treatments, especially when they're experiencing sensitivity or discomfort.

Benefits to Cancer Patients

Polarity therapy promotes healing on all levels, Callinan says. Patients understand more about their bodies from a holistic point of view, and achieve integration that otherwise might be lacking. On a physical level, she says, the treatments help to improve blood and lymph circulation, strengthen the nervous and musculoskeletal systems, and reduce the trauma from stress and disease.

Compatibility with Conventional Treatment

Polarity treatments are completely compatible with cancer treatments, Callinan says. Her clients have reported that they find it easier to tolerate conventional cancer treatments after starting the sessions.

FOR FURTHER INFORMATION

Contact the American Polarity Therapy Association (APTA) at (303) 545-2080 to request a copy of the APTA Members Index, which lists all APP and RPP members by region. The index costs $3.00. Their web site is www.polaritytherapy.org

American Polarity Therapy Association (APTA)
P.O. Box 19858
Boulder, CO 80308

BOOKS RECOMMENDED BY HEALERS

Health Building: The Conscious Art of Living Well. **Randolph Stone** (Reno, Nevada: CRCS Publications, 1985).

ROLFING

Rolfing® is the trademark name for a method of structural integration created by Ida Rolf. Its aim is the realignment of the body by manipulation of the fascia, or connective tissue. Fascia is found throughout the body, surrounding every muscle, bone, and organ, connecting one part of the body to the other.

When fascia is damaged—as a result of surgery, for example—it often hardens, contracts, or adheres to muscles or bone, resulting in pain, a decreased range of motion, and sometimes emotional distress.

The goal of Rolfing is to loosen, lengthen, stretch, and lift the fascia throughout the body, returning the body to a more balanced state.

■ HOW IT HELPS ■

By releasing the fascia and aligning the body to itself and gravity, patients report that they enjoy improved breathing, lessening of chronic pain and stiffness, better mobility and posture, reduced stress, and greater energy.

Because Rolfing involves deep bodywork, it shouldn't be performed for several weeks following cancer surgery. Once the healing process is well under way, however, Rolfing treatments can make a significant difference.

"I recommend Rolfing postoperatively because freeing the fascia around a surgical site results in more freedom and comfort, as well as better healing," says William G. Short, a certified Rolfer and Rolf movement practitioner in Washington, D.C.

■ WHAT TO EXPECT ■

Rolfing sessions usually last about sixty minutes, and patients are often advised to have a series of ten sessions.

During initial sessions, clients are asked about the types and locations of discomfort they may be experiencing. The practitioner will observe the client's movement and posture, and also move the body in different ways to determine whether there are problems with muscle-bone connections, or with the body's connective tissue, which may be contributing to generalized discomfort.

The therapist then will begin treatment on the patient, who typically lies on a massage table. The therapist will apply varying amounts of pressure, usually with the fingers and knuckles, and sometimes with the elbows or knees, in order to stretch connective tissues. Because pressure is applied, treatments can produce discomfort, depending on the individual's condition, but it shouldn't last beyond the treatment. Some patients will have mild stiffness or soreness afterward, but the discomfort usually goes away fairly quickly.

■ TRAINING ■

The Rolf Institute is the approved Rolfing training institution. Training may be completed in 1.5 to 2 years in Boulder, Colorado, or at a satellite program, and is offered in three distinct units. After successful completion of training, and 3 years of practice, the certified Rolfer may continue training to become a certified advanced Rolfer.

Regulation varies considerably by state, as does coverage by health insurance providers. In some states, Rolfing falls under massage practice legislation. A packet on accessing health insurance coverage is available from the Rolf Institute upon request.

■ TREATMENT FROM TOP PRACTITIONERS ■

William G. Short *is a certified Rolfer and Rolf movement practitioner in Washington, D.C., where he has practiced since 1990.*

Treatment Goals

"I look at cancer as a full-body issue, regardless of its origin," Short says. "I've worked part-time for nine years in a psychiatric facility, which has given me a better understanding of, and appreciation for, the mind-body interaction. I look at the connection between cancer and a person's understanding of the mind-body relationship. Dr. Rolf found that by aligning the body with gravity, the healing process could be enhanced."

Rolfing takes into account the ways we use our bodies in our daily lives, Short explains. When people deal with significant trauma, such as a cancer diagnosis, their physical bodies bear the weight of this burden. "Working with a Rolfer can help to improve flexibility, increase range of motion after surgery, and provide supportive touch to nurture the body's own healing abilities," Short says.

Treatment Session

Before beginning any Rolfing work, Short takes a history of past traumas, as well as what has worked well for the person in the past. This discussion can take place either during the initial session or by telephone before meeting.

"I want to help people become aware of their body responses as another resource, as a tool to help them observe how they are doing," Short says. "Together, we monitor physical shifts and changes during each session. These observations of changes, both large and small, provide a kind of road map to help us remain more present to the healing process."

The initial Rolfing process usually requires eight to twelve sessions. Depending on the needs of the client, appointments can be scheduled weekly, monthly, or semimonthly. Each session lasts approximately one hour.

A typical treatment session begins with a few minutes of conversation, assessment, and setting of treatment goals. The client may be asked to stand, turn, and walk while wearing undergarments. The client is then asked to lie on the treatment table for the Rolfing work. Conversations may occur throughout the treatment, as the client is actively involved in the session.

Benefits to Cancer Patients

"Cancer happens over time, and Rolfing works with the whole person over time, taking into account the past as well as the present," Short says. "Rolfing increases a person's ability to adapt to situations; from increasing mobility and flexibility to a greater understanding of how our bodies work and respond to varied situations."

Clients who complete the treatments are better able to handle stress. At the same time, they find they can release old structural patterns and find improved skills to cope with current situations, Short says. It's not uncommon for cancer patients who have the treatments to improve in mobility and range of motion. They may also enhance their recovery after surgery.

Compatibility with Conventional Treatment

There's no reason that Rolfing can't be done in conjunction with standard cancer treatments, Short says. However, he recommends that clients not have Rolfing sessions in the two months following surgery in order to give the body time to heal. He has treated clients during chemotherapy and will work with clients undergoing radiation. In this case, Short adjusts treatment according to the sensitivity of the individual; he coordinates his treatments with the radiation treatment schedule, working closely with his client's radiation oncologist.

FOR FURTHER INFORMATION

Contact the Rolf Institute at (800) 530-8875, or access their web site, www.rolf.org, to obtain a referral listing for certified Rolfers.

The Rolf Institute
205 Canyon Boulevard
Boulder, CO 80302

BOOKS RECOMMENDED BY HEALERS

Ida Rolf Talks About Rolfing and Physical Reality. **Rosemary Feitis (Ed.)** (New York: Harper and Row, 1978).

Rolfing: Reestablishing the Natural Alignment and Structural Integration of the Human Body for Vitality and Well-Being. **Ida P. Rolf (Rochester, Vermont: Healing Arts Press, 1989).**

Rolfing: Stories of Personal Empowerment. **Brian Anson (Kansas City, Missouri: Heartland Personal Growth Press, 1991).**

Spacious Body: Explorations in Somatic Ontology. **Jeffrey Maitland (Berkeley, California: North Atlantic Books,1995).**

SHIATSU

Shiatsu is an ancient healing art from Japan that is based on the principles of traditional Chinese medicine. It employs a sustained pressure applied to specific points along acupuncture meridians to release and disperse blocked energy, or qi. Ideally, one's energy is balanced and flowing freely when in good health. But as our defenses are weakened and resources exhausted, as may be the case for cancer patients, energy flow can be interrupted or thrown out of balance. The goal of shiatsu is to help balance a person's energy to set the conditions for a natural healing process to occur.

■ HOW IT HELPS ■

Shiatsu has long been reported to relax and release stiffness, reduce pain and fatigue, improve energy, promote overall physical and emotional well-being, rejuvenate the mind and body, relieve stress and tension, promote restful sleep, and promote the natural healing process.

Sharon Benoliel, a shiatsu practitioner in Potomac, Maryland, has worked with patients suffering from cancer. "Shiatsu has been very helpful for pain relief and improving a sense of well-being," she says. "It also supports the immune system, while helping the body and mind to heal and function optimally."

There's some evidence that shiatsu can also be used to relieve nausea from chemotherapy. In a study conducted by researchers at the Institute for Health and Aging at the University of California, San Francisco, women undergoing chemotherapy were given treatments that involved putting finger pressure on acupressure points on the forearm and knee.[14] The women who received the treatments had less nausea than those who didn't get the treatments. Even when they did experience nausea, it was less intense than among the nontreatment group.

■ WHAT TO EXPECT ■

Most shiatsu sessions last sixty minutes. After the practitioner takes a health history, the client is usually instructed to lie on a mat or futon while the practitioner uses his or her hands to feel the energy along different meridians. The goal is to detect blockages in the body's energy, and to use hand pressure to release the blockages and allow energy to flow more freely.

Shiatsu sessions are usually performed through a person's clothes. The practitioner will press on specific shiatsu points along different meridians; the pressure can be quite gentle or firm at times, depending on the client's preferences.

If the practitioner determines that the body's energy is extremely deficient or out of balance, a number of sessions may be useful. In other cases, one or two treatments are all that are needed to restore proper energy flow.

■ TRAINING ■

There is no widely accepted standard for shiatsu training. Most programs offered in shiatsu range from one hundred to three hundred hours. There are training and certification programs offered at shiatsu schools around the country. Some massage schools offer shiatsu training as part of their curriculum as well. Most shiatsu practitioners are considered adequately trained after receiving between two hundred and three hundred hours of instruction in shiatsu.

Shiatsu is typically not covered under health insurance. In some states, certified shiatsu practitioners may be regulated by state massage legislation.

■ TREATMENTS FROM TOP PRACTITIONERS ■

Sharon Benoliel *practices at the Shiatsu and Healing Center in Potomac, Maryland. Her certification in ohashiatsu, along with her training in polarity therapy, reiki, and therapeutic touch provides her cancer patients with a rich blend of techniques and skills.*

Treatment Goals

"Shiatsu is used to set the conditions for the body to heal itself," Benoliel says. "I use shiatsu techniques to summon energy to places in most need, and disperse the energy from the areas where it is most congested, thereby restoring the natural flow of energy and reestablishing a state of wellness. It is more similar to acupuncture than massage because it helps to move energy."

Treatment Session

Benoliel sees most clients for seventy-five-minute sessions weekly, although the frequency depends on their needs and preference. She advises them to wear loose clothing because the entire treatment is done with the client fully clothed.

After taking a brief history, she has the patients lie face down, which relaxes them. Then she has them turn over and lie face up, so she can do a diagnostic evaluation, with the emphasis on the abdominal area.

"All of the acupuncture meridians are evaluated," she explains. "The treatment is accomplished by gentle hand pressure at specific points—the shiatsu points—to bring energy back into balance. Usually, when the session is completed, patients feel more relaxed and have more energy. In some cases, they may be tired initially, although they'll have more energy the following day."

Benefits to Cancer Patients

Benoliel views cancer and other diseases as energetic phenomena. Apart from easing pain and improving a sense of well-being, shiatsu helps move a person toward wellness by enhancing the movement of energy along acupuncture meridians, she explains.

Compatibility with Conventional Treatment

Shiatsu is very compatible with conventional cancer therapies, Benoliel says. The treatments are relaxing, and can support an individual emotionally and physically while undergoing standard treatments.

FOR FURTHER INFORMATION

Contact the Associated Bodywork and Massage Professionals, a 34,000-member organization, which provides referrals for over twenty-five different specialties, including shiatsu. Their current listing includes over 1,000 shiatsu practitioners nationwide, who are members of ABMP, licensed practitioners, and have completed a minimum of 100 hours of training at a state-approved school. Their web site is: www.abmp.com, or call ABMP at (800) 458-2267 for a referral.

Associated Bodywork and Massage Professionals
1271 Sugarbush Drive
Evergreen, CO 80439-9766

BOOKS RECOMMENDED BY HEALERS
The Book of Shiatsu. Paul Lundberg
(New York: Simon and Schuster, 1992).

C hiropractic treatment is one of the most popular complementary therapies, used by millions and recognized around the world. In fact, many consider it a mainstream therapy. Spinal adjustments, the cornerstone of chiropractic care, have been practiced from the days of the ancient Egyptians to the present. Chiropractic is one of the largest and fastest growing primary care licensed health care fields in the United States.

This modality's approach to healing is based on the belief that the body can heal itself if proper functioning of the nervous system is restored. This is achieved primarily through alignment of the spine, the gateway to the nervous system. If vertebrae are out of place, and the conduction of nerve impulses is impaired, it can interrupt the normal functioning of other body systems, including organs, bones, muscles, and glands, creating conditions that can lead to disease. Because the nervous system is dependent on proper alignment of the spinal column for optimal functioning, chiropractic focuses on the correction of these misalignments.

■ HOW IT HELPS ■

Chiropractic has been used successfully for certain types of musculoskeletal pain, including lower back pain, headaches, neck pain, and joint and muscle aches. People generally report feeling better after a spinal manipulation, noting such effects as immediate relief from or reduction in pain, improved range of motion, release of tension, and alleviation from general discomfort. Many practitioners as well as patients believe that regular spinal adjustments can be a supportive measure for overall well-being.

Although there have been claims over the years, from chiropractors and patients alike, that chiropractic therapy can affect the outcome of cancer, so far there is no credible scientific evidence to support these claims. There is anecdotal evidence in the literature suggesting that chiropractic may be a useful adjunct treatment to conventional cancer care, reducing pain and the need for pain medication. For cancer patients, chiropractic may be useful in alleviating postsurgical pain and pain associated with radiation, such as fibrosis, or scar adhesions.[15] Nevertheless, chiropractic cannot and should not replace standard medical treatment for cancer. Most practitioners are careful to stress to patients that even though chiropractic can relieve some of the discomforts of cancer or its treatments, it has no effect on the disease itself.

As previously stated, the basic premise of chiropractic is that spinal adjustments can help restore normal neurological function, which in turn improves body functions. Chiropractors theorize that if the spine is in proper alignment, the body will be less encumbered and better able to recover from cancer or any other disease.

"No matter what your condition, you will be better off without nerve damage or imbalance," explains Dr. Marc Smith, a chiropractic neurologist from Gulf Shores, Alabama. Cancer patients often notice that they get a lift, mentally and physically, from the treatments. "With cancer patients, quality of life is often ignored," says Dr. Smith. "Chiropractic handles a lot of the 'aches and pains,' as well the side effects of treatment, such as fatigue, digestive problems, headaches, and hip problems."

Many of the techniques used in chiropractic, including massage and joint and muscle manipulation, have been shown to reduce stress and anxiety as well as muscular pain and tension. In fact, an increasing number of hospitals are now offering chiropractic as part of their services.

It is important to note that although chiropractic care may indeed be of value in maintaining general health and well-being, there are certain conditions in which chiropractic adjustments are contraindicated: for example, fractures, spinal instability, metastatic invasion of bone, advanced osteoporosis, or fever of unknown origin. Therefore, it is particularly important to coordinate your chiropractic care with your medical physician.

■ WHAT TO EXPECT ■

After an initial medical history and physical examination, a treatment plan is offered that usually includes spinal adjustments. As chiropractors are interested in each patient's overall health, additional questions and examinations that target such areas as life stresses, nutrition, and exercise can also be expected.

Spinal adjustments typically consist of a quick, controlled manual thrust. Chiropractors use their hands or an instrument specifically designed for chiropractic use, directed at a very specific location. Using these techniques and tools, chiropractors are often able to restore range of motion and sometimes improve or restore function.

Chiropractic techniques and treatments are varied to meet each patient's needs. Some chiropractic manipulative techniques can be rigorous; other methods use a gentler touch, or slower, constant pressure. Some practitioners use only chiropractic techniques; others may employ additional therapies such as heat, massage, exercise, physical therapy, or even acupuncture. Chiropractors may also refer patients to other practitioners, depending on their needs.

The length and frequency of chiropractic sessions depend on the individual patient's circumstances. Most conditions will be resolved with a limited series of sessions. "Damaged tissue requires at least six to eight weeks to heal properly, so typically we may see someone from six to twelve times or more during that period," says Dr. Smith. In general, initial sessions are from one to two hours in length. Follow-up sessions average fifteen to twenty minutes.

■ TRAINING ■

Doctor of chiropractic applicants must have a minimum of two years of college coursework that meets prechiropractic requirements in order to apply to any of the sixteen nationally accredited chiropractic colleges in the United States. The course of study is four years of full-time resident instruction, and includes an academic and clinical program as well as an internship. Clinical specialty programs include nutrition, child care, neurology, radiology, sports and fitness, and family practice.

MY APPROACH

Peter McPartland, D.C., has been practicing chiropractic for over fifteen years. He currently provides treatment from his office in Silver Spring, Maryland.

"What I look to do is to balance the body's nervous system, thereby allowing the body to better adapt to its environment. As you balance the nervous system, you strengthen the immune system as well. I try to get a patient's life force at its optimum, because in the end, only life can heal. When the body is working at its best, it puts patients in the best position to heal themselves.

"I like to stress that my practice is both high-tech *and* high touch. I am very committed to my role as educator as well as healer, and I require my

All fifty states license chiropractors, and virtually all states will accept applicants for state license who have passed the national boards administered by the National Board of Chiropractic Examiners. Applicants must meet specific state and local requirements for licensure. Almost all states also mandate continuing education on an annual basis to maintain licensure.

Health insurance coverage for chiropractic care is mandated in some states and is available from many insurance carriers.

■ TREATMENT FROM TOP PRACTITIONERS ■

Julie Rosenberg, D.C., *is a board-certified chiropractic neurologist in Rockville, Maryland. About 10 to 15 percent of her clients are cancer survivors.*

Treatment Goals

Chiropractic neurology is a cutting-edge specialty, with fewer than four hundred practitioners in the United States. Dr. Rosenberg uses her additional knowledge and understanding of neuroanatomy and neurophysiology to assess the health and function of a person's nervous sys-

---

patients to attend my lecture on factors that contribute to health, as I believe that chiropractic is only a piece of the puzzle. I want to expand each of my patients' consciousness about how health and healing take place.

"I have found that the survivors I have worked with tend to seek chiropractic treatment for secondary effects from the disease. But regardless of why they seek chiropractic care, I view each patient not symptomatically but holistically, taking into account their physical, spiritual, and emotional health. Treatment has been described as a release, as I believe that healing is a shedding of the illness we have accumulated. My patients have found a decrease in pain, reduction in tightness, and overall lighter feeling, and a feeling of being loved. I believe that my patients leave each session healed on some level, physically, emotionally, or spiritually."

tem. "My specialized training in neurology gives me more tools and allows me to take chiropractic to a deeper level," she says. "I also have a strong background in nutrition, and I combine a number of approaches in helping to restore or enhance a patient's well-being."

Dr. Rosenberg's goal in working with cancer patients is to take as many stressors off the nervous system as possible to allow the immune system and the rest of the body to function optimally while dealing with cancer and cancer treatments. "I can also help with the pain that cancer sometimes brings, so the body can concentrate on what it needs," she says. "I am a strong believer in fixing what I find and letting the body heal itself."

Treatment Session

Dr. Rosenberg's initial session includes a comprehensive examination, a family and medical history, and a review of any recent diagnostic tests. If necessary, she takes blood work or X-rays. This session lasts from one to two hours. Dr. Rosenberg rarely treats patients on the first visit. Instead, she uses the initial session to put together the puzzle pieces. "I look at structure, chemistry, and emotions," she notes. "If one is out of balance, it throws the rest off. I look for the weak link."

After she has collected and reviewed all necessary information, Dr. Rosenberg meets again with the patient to discuss options and begin treatment. Follow-up sessions usually last thirty minutes. Treatment is individualized and includes chiropractic adjustments, recommendations for dietary changes, homeopathy, herbs, vitamins, and nutritional supplements.

Dr. Rosenberg typically sees new patients one or two times a week. Each session usually includes a progress check, treatment, and evaluation. Results are often seen by the fourth or fifth visit. If no changes have been observed after two weeks, she will reevaluate and consider other options. "I am highly committed to getting results, and I ask that my patients share that goal,"she explains.

When discussing reactions to treatments, Dr. Rosenberg notes that her patients often feel different when they leave the office from when they came in. But there are wide variations of reactions to treatments. Dr. Rosenberg has observed that "some patients report feeling lighter overall. Emotional release is not unusual, especially if scar adhesions are being addressed."

Benefits to Cancer Patients

Dr. Rosenberg reports that, in her experience, cancer patients usually feel better after treatments. They may have increased energy, strength, and stamina and decreased pain, and feel more at ease. Emotionally, they may also find that anger and resentment have lessened, they are able to handle things better, and are more at peace with themselves.

Compatibility with Conventional Treatment

Dr. Rosenberg finds her work very compatible with conventional cancer care, observing that "more and more, doctors are open to what I do." She estimates that approximately 25 to 30 percent of her patients are from physician referrals.

FOR FURTHER INFORMATION

The International Chiropractors Association (ICA) is the oldest national chiropractic organization in the world. It provides research, advocacy, and education, and has established standards of ethical, technical, and professional excellence for doctors of chiropractic. The ICA provides referrals to their member chiropractors throughout the country.

Contact them at (800) 423-4690, or access their web site, www.chiro-practic.org.

International Chiropractors Association (ICA)
1110 North Glebe Road, Suite 1000
Arlington, VA 22201

The American Chiropractic Association (ACA), a professional organzi-ation for doctors of chiropractic, also makes referrals to participating ACA members who are licensed chiropractic practitioners and in good standing with licensing boards. Listing is voluntary. Contact the ACA at (800) 986-4636 or visit the web site www.acatoday.com for a list of practitioners in your area.

American Chiropractic Association (ACA)
1701 Clarendon Boulevard
Arlington, VA 22209

E nergy healing embraces a broad range of techniques. The underlying philosophy of these different approaches is that a field of energy exists within and extends beyond the physical parameters of the human body, and is composed of many levels. This energy field serves as a unique blueprint in determining our spiritual, emotional, and physical constitution and well-being. When there is a disruption or congestion in the energy field, an imbalance occurs that, if not corrected, can manifest itself in negative emotional or physical conditions.

Energy healers describe their work as restoring a person's vitality through balancing, cleansing, clearing, repairing, and removing any disruptions or blocks to energy flow. The healer serves as a channel for "universal energy" (the life energy that permeates every living thing) to be received by the client. While energy healing doesn't require full understanding or acceptance, it helps to have an openness on the part of the individual, along with the guidance of a skilled healer, to ensure that the energy offered in a healing session is effectively received.

■ HOW IT HELPS ■

While the medical community has largely dismissed energy healing and very little research has been done to validate the effectiveness of energy work or to explain fully its role in healing, many people believe it can help. Those who have experienced energy treatments report that it's effective at easing stress and anxiety, noting that the therapy results in feelings of warmth, relaxation, clarity, and emotional release. It has been used to reduce fatigue, increase stamina, and deepen one's spiritual and emotional growth. Patients have also used energy healing to help them recover from emotional and physical trauma, relieve pain, and minimize the negative side effects of conventional cancer treatments. Clearly, energy healing isn't a cure for cancer, and its validity as an effective treatment has yet to be scientifically proven, but its reported benefits have led cancer patients to include it in their care as a helpful adjunct to conventional treatments.

■ WHAT TO EXPECT ■

Energy sessions often begin with a brief discussion between the client and healer regarding any issues of concern. The treatments are usually performed on fully clothed clients lying on a massage table. Sessions typically last sixty minutes.

There are many types of energy healing; each style varies somewhat in technique. Four styles profiled here are reiki, therapeutic touch, healing touch, and Brennan Healing Science®.

Reiki

Reiki involves placement of the healer's hands directly on or just above the energy centers of the body, also known as "chakras." The chakras correspond to particular areas of the body, such as the throat, stomach, or heart. Reiki practitioners say they direct the "universal life energy" to where it is needed by the patient. The hands remain still; no massage is involved. Clients can learn to perform reiki on themselves.

Therapeutic Touch

This energy healing treatment was introduced in the 1970s by Dolores Krieger, R.N., Ph.D., and Dora Kunz; it's commonly practiced by nurses. It employs two basic techniques: a sweeping or brushing movement of the hands slightly above the client (used in assessment and clearing), and a still position of the hands, either lightly touching or slightly above the client, to transfer the energy from the "universal source" to the client.

Healing Touch

Healing touch is a more expansive program of energy healing that embraces many types of energy treatments, including therapeutic touch. Healing touch practitioners place their hands both directly on and above the patient, allowing for more variation in movement of the hands and more variation in distance from which the treatment is applied than do other styles of energy healing.

Practitioners are trained to apply particular treatments to specific health conditions or circumstances. For example, a cleansing treatment called magnetic unruffle is used to treat people recovering from general anesthesia.

Brennan Healing Science®

Practitioners from the Barbara Brennan School of Healing® have trained under the direction of Barbara Brennan, a healer, therapist, and former research scientist. These healers are trained in using a wide array of techniques to work on the "human energy consciousness field." Their goal is to integrate the physical, mental, emotional, and spiritual levels of an individual. They employ a direct transmission of energy through their hands to the client, applied anywhere an imbalance, depletion, or blockage is found.

The effects of energy healings can be subtle: some individuals may feel no different physically after experiencing a healing. However, Susan Buell, a certified reiki master teacher in Alexandria, Virginia, reports that many of her clients feel energy immediately in multiple parts of their body. She observes that "usually energy is felt moving slowly and gently from the head to the feet. It is typically very peaceful." Patients have reported experiencing feelings of warmth or heat. Others may feel slightly light-headed or fatigued for a brief period. "They begin to understand their energy and how it feels in different parts of the body, " says Buell.

There is also no reliable prediction of how long an energy healing session will benefit the client, or how many sessions will be needed. Some healers suggest scheduling energy work at specific times during cancer treatment to minimize side effects and support the patient when undergoing certain procedures. Healers will make themselves available to hospitalized patients. Irene Morelli, R.N., has been a therapeutic touch practitioner for more than twenty years. "I love to treat my clients in the recovery room following surgery because my work helps to reduce the side effects from anesthesia," she says.

■ TRAINING ■

Preparation for practicing energy healing varies considerably among the methods described, because comprehensive standards for education, training and certification, and skill levels have not yet been determined. Training can range from self-teaching to weekend workshops to intensive multi-year training and certification programs.

Reiki training can be accomplished in structured workshops or through individual instruction by a reiki master. One can achieve the title of reiki master after a few days training or over a more extended period of time. Several training programs are available throughout the United States, most of which offer all four levels of training. Reiki I, II, and advanced reiki training are required before progressing to reiki master. There is currently no central association or certifying organization for reiki.

Healing touch students can choose from different levels of education depending on the program and the individual's goals. Training can take as much as several years. The Healing Touch International three-level certification program includes weekend and residential courses and a mentoring program for health care professionals and laypersons.

Therapeutic touch, under the direction of Dolores Krieger, R.N., Ph.D., offers three levels of preparation: beginner, intermediate, and advanced. The program is available to nurses, other health care professionals, and laypersons. The Nurse Healers-Professional Associates International (NH-PAI) is the official organization for therapeutic touch and sets the standards for teaching and practice. Most members are health care professionals.

Brennan Healing Science practitioners complete a comprehensive, intensive four-year program of coursework in both healing techniques and self-transformation at the Barbara Brennan School of Healing. Advanced studies and teacher training programs are also offered.

Legislated energy healing regulations are virtually nonexistent. Health insurance coverage is generally not available.

■ TREATMENTS FROM TOP PRACTITIONERS ■
Maureen H. McCracken, R.N., *is a certified healing touch practitioner and instructor. She's also a licensed psychiatric mental health clinical nurse specialist in Herndon, Virginia. In her work with cancer patients, she employs massage as well as psychotherapeutic techniques.*

Treatment Goals

"I support cancer clients in choosing their own path in their healing," McCracken says. "My goal is to work with clients in developing positive life strategies for healing emotionally, mentally, and spiritually."

McCracken helps clients work through issues associated with cancer, such as loss, transition, and marital problems. "My goal in using healing touch is to balance and harmonize a client's energy field, reduce the side effects of allopathic treatment, and increase well-being."

Treatment Session

During the initial visit, McCracken obtains a health history and discusses the client's current situation. A plan of treatment is developed, and goals are established. In subsequent sessions, she uses a variety of techniques—not only healing touch, but also visualization and talk therapy.

MY APPROACH

Betty Caldwell is a certified energy healer and graduate of the Barbara Brennan School of Healing. She treats patients with cancer and other illnesses at her office in Columbia, Maryland, and sees people pre- and postoperatively at Baltimore- and Washington-area hospitals.

"My clients come to me to learn how to live their lives more at peace, in a less anxious way, especially in between those medical check-ups. Through our work, they begin to set new goals and look at their life's purpose. We look at the larger context of their experiences, which helps them regain a sense of influence over what's going on for them.

"I help support the whole person, helping them to transform the physical, emotional, and spiritual aspects of cancer they experience. I support them in their work with allopathic conventional treatment, bringing additional relief, knowledge, energy, and tools for self-healing.

"I work with an array of healing tools, including direct transmission of energy through my hands, as well as selected therapeutic essential oils and flower essences to help move clients forward in their healing.

McCracken has her clients lie on a massage table, fully clothed. Healing touch can be done hands-on or hands-off, depending on client preference. McCracken usually begins at the head, moving down the body as she removes energy blocks and balances and cleanses all the layers of energy that compose the auric field. In addition, interactive guided imagery is used during healing touch treatments.

McCracken also uses prayer in her sessions. "Working with a person's spiritual system, I recommend prayer because I feel it's very important to healing."

The sessions last forty-five minutes. Clients are seen weekly at first. Individualized schedules evolve as needs are identified and the client's reaction to the energy work is defined.

Reactions to healing touch commonly include mood elevation and tension reduction. "Most people tell me

---

"Most people find the treatments very relaxing, supportive, and energizing. I have found that energy healing helps with radiation fatigue, pain relief, and relaxation. Pain relief is common, and many of my clients tell me our work has had an impact on how they view their experience. I have seen patients lessen their experience with chronic illness and improve their general health. It is also valuable in dealing with the emotional and spiritual issues surrounding cancer.

"Energy healing is complementary to allopathic cancer treatment, and I recommend the two be used in conjunction with each other. I also try to schedule energy sessions as soon after a chemotherapy treatment as possible, and offer energy support during radiation treatments, prior to surgery, during actual surgery (if approved by the physician), and postoperatively.

"I have had good relationships with physicians in the past, and I'm more than willing to work with clients' doctors. In fact, I will only see cancer clients who are being treated by a physician, whether they have chosen a conventional or unconventional treatment program."

they find it really uplifting. To feel spiritually upheld and supported is a really important thing," says McCracken.

Benefits to Cancer Patients

McCracken reports that her work helps alleviate depression, anxiety, and pain; decreases side effects of chemotherapy, radiation, and surgery; increases feelings of well-being; and increases optimism and spiritual growth.

Compatibility with Conventional Treatment

The treatments are compatible with standard medical treatments for cancer, McCracken says. In fact, she advises patients to schedule healing touch treatments in conjunction with chemotherapy. "If someone receives a treatment just prior to chemotherapy, it is generally better tolerated," she says. "If a treatment is given just after chemotherapy, side effects are often reduced."

FOR FURTHER INFORMATION
Contact the following organizations:

The International Center for Reiki Training
21421 Hilltop Street, Unit 28
Southfield, MI 48034
(800) 332-8112
www.reiki.org, for a list of reiki teachers.

Healing Touch International
12477 West Cedar Drive, Suite 202
Lakewood, CO 80228
(303) 989-7982
www.healingtouch.net, for a list of over 1,200 certified healing touch practitioners.

Nurse Healers-Professional Associates International
3760 South Highland Drive, Suite 429
Salt Lake City, UT 84106
(801) 273-3399

Access the web site, www.therapeutic-touch.org, for referrals to therapeutic touch practitioners worldwide and recommended literature on
therapeutic touch.

The Barbara Brennan School of Healing
500 Northeast Spanish River Boulevard, Suite 108
Boca Raton, FL 33431
(561) 620-8767
Call (800) 924-2564 or access their web site,
www.barbarabrennan.com, for an international directory of their
practitioners.

BOOKS RECOMMENDED BY HEALERS

*The Complete Reiki Handbook: Basic Introduction and Methods of Natural
Application: A Complete Guide for Reiki Practice.* **Walter Lübeck (Twin Lakes,
Wisconsin: Lotus Press, 1998).**

Empowerment Through Reiki: The Path to Personal and Global Transformation.
Paula Horan (Twin Lakes, Wisconsin: Lotus Press, 1992).

*Hands of Light: A Guide to Healing Through the Human Energy Field: A New
Paradigm for the Human Being in Health, Relationship and Disease.* **Barbara Ann
Brennan (Toronto, New York: Bantam Books, 1988).**

Light Emerging: The Journey of Personal Healing. **Barbara Ann Brennan (New
York: Bantam Books, 1993).**

Therapeutic Touch: A Practical Guide. **Janet Macrae (New York: Knopf,
1988).**

HOLISTIC COUNSELING AND PSYCHOTHERAPY:
Self-Regulation Techniques

For some time, counseling and psychotherapy have been recognized as important adjunctive therapies for cancer patients. The benefits of these modalities have long been proven and accepted in our culture; physicians often recommend that their patients seek such counseling services while undergoing medical treatment or as they learn to adjust to cancer as part of their lives.

Counseling can be a valuable component of any integrated treatment plan, for two reasons. First, emotional healing is vital to the total health of a human being, and it's a critical component of the holistic model used in complementary cancer care. Second, some traditional psychotherapists today are embracing many techniques that until now have been considered alternatives.

Social workers and psychotherapists are supplementing their "talk" therapies with complementary techniques that have a powerful impact on emotional support and healing. For instance, Martha Bramhall, L.C.S.W.-C., trained as a clinical social worker and practicing in Silver Spring, Maryland, now calls herself a spiritually oriented psychotherapist. In an article published in the *Society for Spirituality and Social Work* newsletter, she explains that her evolution toward a more holistic practice has been based in part on her belief that "we each sit on the three-legged stool of body, mind, and spirit. If we are to heal our wounds of the past or become more integrated or complete, it is necessary to strengthen each leg of the stool. It is within the realm of psychotherapy to work with each facet."

Like Ms. Bramhall, many therapists are expanding their work by blending complementary approaches and mind-body techniques with their standard professional training to provide holistic services that are unique. There now seem to be as many combinations of therapies, treatment tools, techniques, and approaches as there are practitioners. Along with talk therapy, a practice might include a combination of yoga, energy work, guided imagery, sound therapy, biofeedback, or color therapy, to name a few. Many of the services being offered are actually self-care tools that enable clients to help themselves.

Described here are two of the more widely used complementary techniques, popular with people living with cancer, that are often included as part of holistic counseling and psychotherapy practices.

BIOFEEDBACK

The word "biofeedback," when broken down, describes exactly what this treatment provides. With the use of monitoring instruments, individuals are given immediate insight into their own biology. Biofeedback allows them to actually alter some of their physical responses and feel more in control of their health. They can learn to consciously control what are normally considered involuntary physiological responses, such as skin temperature, heart rate, muscle tension, respiration, or brain waves. Training in biofeedback helps patients to be more aware of their bodies, and they can gain a better understanding of how the mind and the body work in conjunction to heal the individual.

Judith Nelson Siegel, a licensed clinical social worker, practices biofeedback, biofeedback-assisted psychotherapy, and other mind-body treatments in Chevy Chase, Maryland. She has observed that "individuals dealing with cancer have a lot of fear and confusion about their own bodies." She explains that with biofeedback and psychotherapy, the emphasis is on self-awareness and self-regulation, helping clients to develop a greater awareness of and voluntary control over their physiological and psychological processes. " I see my clients develop a sense of control and self-confidence that can be applied throughout their lives," says Siegel. "During the process, clients develop a profound sense of themselves. Clients learn that they can affect their own physiology quickly. This experience often has a powerful and rich effect."

■ HOW IT HELPS ■

Practitioners use biofeedback to ease many physical and emotional problems that are common among cancer patients, including side effects from chemotherapy, insomnia, pain, depression, headaches, stress, fatigue, gastrointestinal disorders, and muscular dysfunction. Biofeedback can also promote profound feelings of relaxation and reduce muscular tension.

Scientific studies have supported a connection between biofeedback and improved immune response. As far back as 1988, studies involving breast cancer patients showed significant positive changes in immune system response after patients received biofeedback.[16, 17] "Recent research shows that balanced brain function is a major player in helping the immune system to regain its proper function," says Mary Lee Esty, Ph.D., a licensed social worker and biofeedback practitioner in Chevy Chase, Maryland. "Biofeedback and neurofeedback act as guides for evaluating and modifying your own physiology. Healthy balanced brain function results in better energy and mood, and is basic to good health."

Research has also shown that biofeedback, by allowing patients to exert control over their breathing rate, is a powerful technique for relieving stress. It's normal, for example, for people to experience shallow, rapid breathing when they're anxious—prior to receiving chemotherapy, for example. With biofeedback, patients are able to monitor their breathing while practicing stress-reduction techniques, such as visualization or meditation. With practice they can learn to slow and deepen their breathing "on command," which floods the tissues with oxygen and helps relieve emotional and physical stress.

Biofeedback has proven to be effective in relieving pain, a common—and sometimes debilitating—problem for cancer patients. Once they learn biofeedback from a skilled practitioner, patients find they can reduce muscle tension and cope with pain more readily. The American Society of Anesthesiologists, in practice guidelines for cancer pain management, calls for the use of biofeedback or other psychosocial interventions as an adjunct to treatment with analgesics.

■ WHAT TO EXPECT ■

A biofeedback session is painless and noninvasive. It involves sitting comfortably while the therapist attaches electrodes to the skin at various points. The patient is asked to divide his or her attention between some form of relaxation, such as visualization or meditation, and focusing on a desired change in a particular body function.

While observing a computer screen or listening for an auditory signal, patients are able to see or hear any changes in physiological measurements that result from changes in their behavior or thoughts. Overall, biofeedback treatment is a relaxing experience, particularly if you keep in mind that it is also a learning experience. As with any type of training, it may take time before significant improvements are noted. Patients learn to associate changes they can make with a more positive outcome for their condition; over time, they can employ biofeedback as a self-healing technique.

If you decide to pursue biofeedback, keep in mind that there are several types. According to *The Alternative Medicine Handbook*, these include:

- Electromyography (EMG). It measures muscle tension, and is used to treat muscular pain and injury and incontinence.
- Thermal. It measures skin temperature, and is used to treat headaches, anxiety, and circulatory conditions.
- Electrodermal (EDA). It measures changes in perspiration, and is used to treat anxiety.
- Respiration and pulse feedback. It is used to treat anxiety and hyperventilation (rapid breathing).

Another kind of biofeedback is the electroencephalogram (EEG), or neurofeedback. It monitors brain wave activity, and is useful in treating depression, anxiety, stress, insomnia, chronic fatigue, and chronic pain.

A relatively new, advanced form of biofeedback therapy called the Flexyx Neurotherapy System™ involves using the patient's own brainwaves to help determine the feedback to the brain to "correct" imbalances in the distribution of energy in the EEG. There is no conscious learning required of the patient. It is used to treat brain injury, extreme stress, post-traumatic stress disorder, anxiety, depression, emotional trauma, and fibromyalgia.

■ TRAINING ■

Many biofeedback practitioners are licensed psychotherapists or counselors trained in biofeedback, but other health professionals such as nurses and physical therapists offer biofeedback therapy as part of their services as well.

The Biofeedback Certification Institute of America (BCIA) offers two certification programs: EEG or neurofeedback, and general biofeedback, such as muscle tension and temperature training. A bachelor's degree in a BCIA-approved health care field is a prerequisite. Certification requirements include specific didactic education, a specified number of supervised practice hours, and a written examination. Certification is voluntary, and for those who are certified, recertification is required every four years. Insurance coverage for biofeedback varies by state, company, and diagnosis.

■ **TREATMENTS FROM TOP PRACTITIONERS** ■

Lilian Rosenbaum, Ph.D., *practices individual and family psychotherapy and biofeedback in Chevy Chase, Maryland. She has been in practice for more than thirty years.*

MY APPROACH

Mary Lee Esty, Ph.D., is a licensed social worker and biofeedback practitioner in Chevy Chase, Maryland. She's also certified in hypnosis and neurofeedback.

"One of the goals of biofeedback is to help clients find their way back to a balanced state, so that the immune system functions better. Biofeedback also helps relieve the depression, fatigue, and cognitive problems that frequently occur following chemotherapy. I try to help patients find a new way of being with their bodies, and to feel some control.

"I use EEG biofeedback in my practice. Using advanced computer technology, electrodes are attached to various parts of the head to obtain a map of the brainwaves. Once the mapping is completed, I discuss with the patient whether this treatment is appropriate. If it is, I estimate how many sessions are needed to achieve the individual's goals.

"Patients are always in control of the biofeedback process. A lot of people think biofeedback is done *to* someone. But in actuality, you do

Treatment Goals

In her practice, Dr. Rosenbaum coaches people with cancer on how best to manage the illness, heal, and enhance their quality of life.

"Biofeedback is one of many components for healing, along with nutrition, exercise, and prayer," Rosenbaum says. "Biofeedback helps people learn to observe and change their own physiological signals to help regulate some aspects of their bodies, thoughts, behavior, and relationships." Rosenbaum notes that biofeedback can also be used by the patient's families and caregivers to manage stress.

Treatment Session

"Most of my cancer patients come to me looking for something to help them get through their medical treatments, something that will strengthen and calm them,"

---

biofeedback to yourself, taking it as far as you want to. The practitioner serves as the coach.

"Cancer patients often report improvements with mood, cognitive functioning, and energy; they also may experience a greater sense of ease and clarity. As people learn certain techniques, they can change their immune system, improving their quality of life. It seems paradoxical, but cancer patients often tell me that they believe that their cancer is one of the greatest things to happen to them. In part this may be because biofeedback has led them to greater self-awareness, self-control, and a deeper connection to the soul. Patients develop greater acceptance of some things, resolution of others, and new priorities and values.

"Biofeedback is completely compatible with conventional treatments. I help prepare people for surgery with biofeedback and guided imagery. I am seeing more physician interest in biofeedback and imagery, as well as more referrals. Many medical centers are now requiring the use of imagery tapes prior to surgery because of the powerful positive impact that it has on healing."

Rosenbaum says. "Often, they want to learn to do something specific with biofeedback."

In the first session, she helps clients get a broader view of what's going on for them and within the family. She often begins by performing computerized monitoring to measure their physiological responses. Then she explains how a patient might benefit from biofeedback.

The initial session lasts fifty to sixty minutes. Subsequent sessions may include a combination of biofeedback and psychotherapy. There is no established schedule for treatment. "They come as often as they wish, depending on their motivation and what is going on in their lives," she says.

Benefits to Cancer Patients

"Biofeedback is used to help enhance the immune system and reduce the stress associated with diagnosis and treatment," Rosenbaum explains. "It also helps in dealing with pain and facilitates more comfortable management of treatments such as radiation and chemotherapy."

Many of Dr. Rosenbaum's patients report that they appreciate the fact that biofeedback allows them to do something for themselves physiologically. Soon after starting treatment, they often report being physiologically calmer and better able to decide about their health care options. Patients have also noted that biofeedback often facilitates the practice of imagery, another self-healing technique.

Compatibility with Conventional Treatment

Rosenbaum has designed her treatment to be compatible with standard cancer treatment. Rosenbaum says, "I ask my clients to sign a release form that allows me to be in communication with their physicians and other health professionals so I can coordinate with their health care team."

FOR FURTHER INFORMATION:

The BCIA provides a geographical list of certified biofeedback practitioners and guidance on selecting practitioners. To receive their information, send a stamped, self-addressed business envelope to BCIA, or access their web site, www.BCIA .org.

The Biofeedback Certification Institute of America

10200 West 44th Avenue, Suite 310

Wheat Ridge, CO 80033

(303) 420-2902

Information on the Flexyx Neurotherapy System can be obtained from the web site www.flexyx.com.

BOOKS RECOMMENDED BY HEALERS

Principles and Practice of Stress Management. Paul M. Lehrer and Robert L. Woolfolk (Eds.) (New York: Guilford Press, 1993).

IMAGERY

Like biofeedback, the practice of imagery is based on the belief that the mind influences our physical health. Also called "guided imagery," this technique involves tapping into the imagination to communicate with the subconscious to help the body and mind to heal. Imagery has helped cancer patients ease pain, distract themselves from their worries, and achieve relaxation and a sense of peace and harmony.

Imagery is the practice of invoking mental images using any or all of our senses. Imagery opens us to the "inner landscape" of our body's experience; it can act as the connector between the voices of our mind, spirit, and body, bringing them together for our physical and emotional well-being.

■ HOW IT HELPS ■

Imagery is a powerful tool that is easily learned, can affect many aspects of our healing, and is valued in part for its versatility. It can be applied to almost any health condition and to many life situations, including cancer, chronic pain, grief, and loss.

Imagery is sometimes incorporated into traditional psychotherapy; it's also used as an adjunct to medical treatment. Specifically with cancer patients, imagery is credited with lessening some of the side effects of conventional treatment—such as anticipatory nausea and vomiting associated with chemotherapy—and improving immune system functioning. Apart from its role in relieving physical discomfort and stress, imagery can help people cope with diseases and difficult life situations by facilitating changes in outlook and attitude, and assisting in preparing for or rehearsing a situation or desired outcome. It can be a valuable tool in decision-making, helping cancer patients to access their intuition, leading to a greater insight and understanding of their illness.

"Imagery helps people open to the spiritual level of facing a disease," says Marilyn Saunders, Ph.D., a counselor who practices imagery therapy in Bethesda, Maryland. "Even if the process does not result in a cure, some patients are able to come to acceptance and experience meaningful inner peace."

Imagery exercises are not only versatile in their application but also in their approach. For instance, when imagery is used for stress relief, it frequently involves imagining a peaceful scene, such as sitting on a beach and listening to the soothing sounds of waves. A more active form of visualization used by cancer patients is to visualize mobilizing the immune system to attack their cancer.

It's not surprising that visualizing peaceful images can lower levels of stress and relieve pain. Studies have shown that patients who fixate on negative, stressful thoughts have an increase in body chemicals (such as adrenaline) that can increase levels of stress as well as depression. Conversely, imagining peaceful, harmonious images causes the body to release soothing chemicals that are similar in structure to sedative medications.

In a study of ninety-four cancer patients receiving bone marrow transplants, published in the medical journal *Pain*, researchers found that those who practiced guided imagery reported less pain than those who didn't. The researchers concluded that imagery is a "powerful component of persistent pain treatment."[18] Some medical centers have included imagery and other self-regulation techniques in comprehensive pain programs.

Although there's no evidence that imagery can result in the destruction of cancer cells, research has shown that imagery can benefit cancer patients in a variety of ways: in addition to relieving pain and lessening the need for pain medication, imagery can lessen anxiety in general as well as that associated with planned medical procedures, and can reduce recovery time from procedures. For instance, a study of 130 colorectal surgical patients conducted by the Cleveland Clinic showed that guided imagery reduced anxiety, pain, the use of pain medication, and length of hospitalization.[19]

Imagery has been proven to be an effective tool in managing pain and contributing to improved immune system functioning. It can be a valuable asset to cancer patients in coping with many of the issues associated with cancer treatment.

■ WHAT TO EXPECT ■

Imagery involves being in what is known as an altered state of consciousness, in which you are in a relaxed state, but awake and aware of your surroundings. This state facilitates access to our inner reality and intuition, bringing us to our body's truth.

When you see a guided imagery practitioner, you'll be taught a variety of different exercises. Most likely you'll be advised to close your eyes and focus on your breathing to induce relaxation, remove distractions, and turn your attention inward.

The practitioner assists in suggesting images to use. Patients are also taught how to bring forth their own images and interact with them to assist the healing process. After learning the technique, imagery can be practiced without professional supervision, sometimes with the use of audiotapes or "scripts" found in books. One advantage of imagery is that it can be practiced anywhere, and at multiple times throughout the day.

■ TRAINING ■

Licensed health professionals can receive training through certification programs or well-established workshops conducted by recognized leaders in the field. The Academy of Guided Imagery, formed in 1989, is an organization that provides training in Interactive Guided Imagery[SM] to health professionals. Training includes 150 hours of independent study and direct supervision over one to two years. The program is accredited by the American Psychological Association. Other training programs are available as well for professionals and laypersons.

Imagery is not licensed in any of the 50 states. Insurance coverage may be available within the practice of a credentialed mental health professional. Imagery work can uncover deep emotions that are best handled in the context of a therapeutic relationship; therefore, it is recommended that imagery be learned and/or practiced with a licensed mental health professional experienced in imagery.

■ TREATMENTS FROM TOP PRACTITIONERS ■

Marilyn Saunders, Ph.D., *of Bethesda, Maryland, is a licensed clinical professional counselor and a founding member of the Imagery Training Institute. She has been in private practice since 1978.*

Treatment Goals

For more than twenty years, Saunders has used imagery as a complement to more traditional talk psychotherapy. She feels that it's a useful tool to help patients integrate mind, body, and spirit.

For cancer patients, Saunders uses imagery to help them understand, literally or metaphorically, what the cancer looks like; what (if any) message it has for them; what their treatment is doing; and how their body is responding.

"My goal in working with cancer clients is to help them claim more of their own inner wisdom and develop their own healing images," Saunders says. "It's important that they relate what's going on in their bodies to what's going on in their lives."

Treatment Session

Saunders uses the initial session to get a sense of the client's present situation, through both talking and an introduction to imagery. Often, images are discovered in the initial session that are appropriate for the client to continue with at home.

Subsequent weekly sessions involve assessing what is happening in the clients' imagery work and in their life, expanding and deepening the imagery work, and suggesting appropriate homework. Usually, Saunders recommends that each client do imagery on his or her own for a few minutes several times a day. Clients are welcome to bring tape recorders to sessions.

Saunders also recommends—and provides—image relationship therapy for the client and his or her partner. She feels that it's important for both people to deal with the stress that illness places on a relationship.

Benefits to Cancer Patients

Saunders reports that those who practice imagery claim more of their own inner wisdom, feel more empowered, and gain a sense of control. "Imagery can help cancer patients make whatever changes are called for." Saunders has observed that those who participate in groups find support for their imagery process and companionship on their journey. "They learn more about receiving from, as well as giving to, others. As the group works with imagery together, it can develop its own metaphorical language, leading to deeper connection and support," she adds.

Compatibility with Conventional Treatment

Imagery is entirely compatible with conventional treatment, and is a good adjunct to it. According to Saunders, by discovering and developing images of what is happening in the body, how the treatment is affecting the cancer, and how the body is responding to the treatment, patients can accept treatment as a true ally rather than a threat to the body. This often results in reduced side effects from treatments, including chemotherapy and radiation.

FOR FURTHER INFORMATION:

Contact the Academy of Guided Imagery at (800)726-2070, or access their web site, www.interactiveimagery.com, for a directory of certified imagery practitioners. The Academy has tapes and books for sale on imagery self-care for the general public, as well as tapes for professionals.

Academy for Guided Imagery

P.O. Box 2070

Mill Valley, CA 94942

(415) 389-9324

BOOKS RECOMMENDED BY HEALERS

(Additional resources for ordering tapes, which include imagery tapes, are included in the Appendix.)

Choices in Healing: Integrating the Best of Conventional and Complementary Approaches to Cancer. Michael Lerner (Cambridge, Massachusetts: MIT Press, 1994). Provides an excellent description of psychotherapeutic approaches, including imagery, to cancer.

Getting Well Again: A Step-by-Step, Self-Help Guide to Overcoming Cancer for Patients and Their Families. O. Carl Simonton, Stephanie Matthews-Simonton, and James Creighton (Los Angeles: J.P. Tarcher; New York: Distributed by St. Martin's Press, 1978).

Healing Yourself: A Step-By-Step Program for Better Health Through Imagery. Martin L. Rossman (New York: Walker, 1987).

Minding the Body, Mending the Mind. Joan Borysenko (Toronto, New York: Bantam Books, 1988).

Rituals of Healing: Using Imagery for Health and Wellness. Jeanne Achterberg, Barbara Dossey, and Leslie Kolkmeier. (New York: Bantam Books, 1994).

Staying Well with Guided Imagery. Belleruth Naparstek (New York: Warner Books, 1994). (Naparstek's *Health Journeys* Guided Imagery Audiotapes are listed in the Appendix.)

Using Imagery in Therapy: A Path to Nurturance, Empowerment and Reconciliation. Marilyn Saunders and Gretchen McKnew (1992). Available through the author: msaunders@peoplepc.com, or www.skillsforthe21stcentury.com, or by calling Lifepath Health Center: (301) 897-8090.

Homeopathy has been an alternative to conventional medicine since its beginnings in the late 1700s. In the United States, homeopathy is sometimes perceived as "fringe" medicine, but it's worth remembering that it's used by millions both here and abroad, and is particularly popular in Europe. For instance, in Britain, homeopathic remedies are covered by the National Health Service. Most French pharmacies offer homeopathic remedies, and approximately 30 to 40 percent of French physicians prescribe homeopathy to their patients.

The therapy's foundation rests on the principle that "like cures like."Samuel Hahnemann, a German physician and the founder of homeopathy, studied many substances—plants, minerals, chemicals, and animal products—for their potential healing qualities. He identified substances that induced symptoms associated with particular illnesses, and then diluted the substances to a miniscule fraction of their original potency, prescribing them to patients suffering from those conditions. His belief was that the diluted remedy could mobilize the immune system to address the illness or condition adequately, much like a vaccine.

The preparation of homeopathic remedies involves many cycles of dilution, in which the substance is extracted from its original source and diluted (usually with water), then shaken vigorously. The process is repeated so many times that most remedies contain none of the molecules from the original substance.

How homeopathy works is still under debate. One theory suggests that the medium containing the essence of the original substance may hold an electromagnetic "message" or "memory" that matches the electromagnetic pattern of the illness. This in turn may activate the body's innate healing capabilities. Similar in principle to vaccines, homeopathic remedies are usually unrelated to the causative agent of the disease, whereas vaccines are derived from the same or a very similar causative agent.

■ HOW IT HELPS ■

Homeopathy is believed to promote overall health, stimulating the body's natural healing responses. Many people in general use homeopathic remedies to help cope with minor illnesses and chronic conditions like colds, earaches, or seasonal allergies, finding they have fewer symptoms and often a faster recovery. For cancer patients, homeopathy has been perceived as being supportive in dealing with the burden of cancer, by helping to cope with side effects from treatment as well as minor illnesses and conditions that can place additional stress on the immune system.

Controversy continues to follow homeopathy, even though its use is on the rise in this country and remains strong elsewhere. Credible scientific studies have shown the efficacy of homeopathic treatment, but a considerable number of research studies dismiss homeopathy as no more than a placebo. And although there have been reports from homeopathic doctors claiming to have successfully treated cancer, these claims are dubious at best.

Although there is little research that clearly demonstrates the benefits of homeopathy for specific conditions, some studies have supported the general effectiveness of homeopathy. For instance, a meta-analysis reported in the *British Medical Journal* reviewed 107 studies of homeopathic medicines. The researchers found that 81 of the studies, or 77 percent, showed positive effects. Of the 22 "best" studies—those designed according to strict scientific criteria—the researchers found that 15 studies, or 68 percent, showed the treatments to be effective.[20]

Most homeopathic remedies are sold without a prescription because they have virtually no side effects and are typically considered safe, although it is not unusual for some people to experience what is known as a healing reaction, in which symptoms are aggravated temporarily. Many have found these remedies to be a useful way to address nagging problems like colds, headaches, or general aches and pains. Homeopathic remedies can often be found in pharmacies and natural food stores. The Food and Drug Administration supervises approval of homeopathic remedies via the *Homeopathic Pharmacopoeia of the United States.*

Cancer patients have turned to homeopathy to alleviate nausea and certain types of pain, reduce anxiety, and increase energy and overall feelings of well-being. For instance, one common symptom in cancer patients is joint pain, a common side effect of cancer treatment. People suffering from chronic arthritis pain have benefited from homeopathic treatment.

Homeopathy may also be helpful in easing skin irritation following radiation treatments, a condition called radiodermatitis. In a study of sixty-six patients who had undergone radiation treatments for breast cancer, researchers found that those who took homeopathic belladonna experienced greater reductions in skin heat than those treated with placebo.[21] Homeopathy can indeed be useful in self-care for minor conditions, and so it can be a good place to start in alleviating those ailments that put additional stress on the body.

Although homeopathy may be a helpful adjunct in treating some of the side effects of cancer and cancer treatments and is considered safe, cancer patients should not depend on it to replace conventional cancer care. There is concern among physicians that patients will avoid seeking necessary medical treatment if they pursue homeopathy as their primary treatment modality.

■ WHAT TO EXPECT ■

Homeopathic treatment addresses the whole patient, and is very specific to the individual. The homeopath gathers information beyond the presenting symptoms, such as underlying minor issues and past health conditions, any physical signs of disease, and the patient's mental state and general emotional makeup. Detailed information on all the qualities of the presenting condition is gathered. This is done in order to identify which single remedy or combination of remedies best matches the client's symptoms and can address the particular situation.

There are more than two thousand substances currently considered to be homeopathic remedies; of these, approximately 200 are commonly used. When you see a homeopath, he or she will recommend specific remedies, in either pill or liquid form, which are typically taken daily, up to several times a day, until the condition or symptoms are resolved.

■ TRAINING ■

In this country, homeopathy is most commonly practiced by licensed health care providers under their primary specialty. According to the National Center for Homeopathy, certification to practice homeopathic medicine is available to M.D.s and D.O.s through the American Board of Homeotherapeutics, to N.D.s through the Homeopathic Academy of Naturopathic

Physicians, and to other professionals through the Council for Homeopathic Certification.

The Council on Homeopathic Education (CHE) is the recognized authority regarding the quality of education provided to licensed professionals. Three U.S. naturopathic colleges (in Washington, Oregon, and Arizona) offer CHE-approved four-year programs leading to an N.D. degree that include extensive coursework in homeopathy. Several multiyear, part-time, and home study programs offer professional and nonprofessional training in homeopathy to health care practitioners and lay persons.

Arizona, Connecticut, and Nevada have state licensing laws specific to homeopathy for M.D.s and/or D.O.s. Currently, naturopathic physicians, trained in homeopathy as well as other natural health modalities, are licensed in eleven states to diagnose and treat illness. Other health care providers may use homeopathy within the scope of their primary licensed practice in the state in which they reside. It is important to be informed about homeopathic and/or naturopathic regulations in your state and especially prudent to familiarize yourself with the qualifications and credentials of any homeopathic practitioners you are considering working with. Medical physicians who are board-certified in homeopathy use the initials D.Ht.; naturopaths use D.H.A.N.P., and other professionals (such as nurse practitioners or acupuncturists) use C.C.H.

Some health insurance companies provide reimbursement for homeopathic services administered by licensed physicians under their primary health specialty.

■ TREATMENTS FROM TOP PRACTITIONERS ■

David Wember, M.D., D.Ht., *is a licensed physician in Rockville, Maryland, who has practiced homeopathy for over twenty-five years.*

Treatment Goals

Dr. Wember explains his orientation is toward treating the patient instead of the disease.

"Although I have treated many people with cancer, I do not treat cancer directly. I try to determine the nature of what is going on for the patients and how their symptoms affect them in order to find a homeopathic remedy that will move them back into balance."

Treatment Session

An initial visit with Dr. Wember lasts approximately one hour and involves an extensive history of present symptoms, medical history, family history, and general constitutional history. Dr. Wember also asks questions to determine what affects patients in their environment. "I want to know what makes their symptoms better or worse, what side of the body the symptoms are on, and how they are affected by the seasons or temperature," he explains. "I look at a patient's general nature as well as particular cravings such as thirsts or cravings for foods." All of this information helps Dr. Wember to find the right homeopathic formula that is individually effective for a patient.

Usually a homeopathic remedy is prescribed at the first visit. For cancer patients, nutritional supplements and diet are recommended and a follow-up remedy is prescribed for related complaints. A second visit is typically scheduled in three to six weeks to evaluate the effectiveness of the treatment plan. Dr. Wember notes that there are no side effects to homeopathic remedies; however, some remedies may cause symptoms to get worse temporarily before the patient gets better, others may provide immediate improvement.

Benefits to Cancer Patients

According to Dr. Wember, homeopathic remedies can be

helpful in reducing the side effects of chemotherapy, helping patients to tolerate the chemotherapeutic drugs better
without interfering with their effectiveness. The remedies
are especially helpful with the nausea and vomiting that
can accompany cancer treatments. According to Dr.
Wember, homeopathic medicine also works to strengthen
the immune system and improve a patient's sense of well-
being.

Compatibility with Conventional Treatment

Dr. Wember reports that homeopathy is very compatible
with conventional treatment and does not interfere with
allopathic medication. "In fact, I do not take patients off
of any medications that have been prescribed and I want
all of my patients to be followed by an allopathic physician. As they begin to feel better, they can talk to their
physician about reducing their medication. I also refer to
many kinds of doctors so that nothing is missed."

FOR FURTHER INFORMATION

The American Board of Homeotherapeutics publishes a directory of
certified homeopaths. To order a copy, contact The National Center for
Homeopathy at (703) 548-7790 and visit their web site for information
on homeopathy and selecting a qualified homeopath: www.homeopath-
ic.org.

National Center for Homeopathy
801 North Fairfax, Suite 306
Alexandria, VA 22314

The Homeopathic Academy of Naturopathic Physicians provides a listing
by state of their members. Visit their web site, www.healthy.net/hanp, to
view their referrals, or contact them at (208) 336-3390.

The Homeopathic Academy of Naturopathic Physicians
1412 West Washington Street
Boise, ID 83702

BOOKS RECOMMENDED BY HEALERS

Discovering Homeopathy: Medicine for the 21st Century. **Dana Ullman**
(Berkeley: North Atlantic Books, 1991).

Healing with Homeopathy: The Complete Guide.
Wayne B. Jonas and Jennifer Jacobs (New York: Warner Books, 1996).

MEDITATIVE PRACTICES

Meditative practices include a number of modalities, including meditation, yoga, and qi gong. Each of these techniques places great value on breathing and breathwork, balance, alignment, and "mindfulness," which means being fully in the present moment. Many students have also found that these practices serve as a means to deepening their spiritual growth.

Cancer patients have long been attracted to meditative practices. Some of the reasons are obvious. Cancer is among the most stressful life experiences people face, and the regular use of meditation, yoga, or other calming practices has been shown to reduce levels of stress and anxiety dramatically. What people often fail to realize is that meditation and related disciplines can also have a profound effect on the physiological manifestations of disease—everything from pain and nausea to the ability of the immune system to recognize and destroy abnormal cells.

All meditative practices are considered to be "self-healing," which means that you can use them to cultivate your inner healing powers. Meditative practices can be self-taught (through videos, audiotapes, or books), although they're preferably learned from a teacher. Once learned, they can also be practiced by the individual without the presence or intervention of a teacher.

Practices can be tailored to the individual, and can be done in solitude or in a group. Most can be done by people of any age or physical condition. There is enough variety in these practices to allow for individual needs and circumstances. Few "tools" or props are necessary; usually the only requirement is your conscious awareness. All have enjoyed great devotion by many people for many years.

MEDITATION

Practiced for thousands of years and popular around the world, meditation has a certain aura of mystery attached to it. It is common for people in our culture to be somewhat awed by meditation, believing they will never be able to understand it fully or to practice it correctly.

It's true that some practitioners of meditation devote many hours to mastering different techniques, but it doesn't have to be time-consuming or difficult. Mediation can simply be an activity that allows you to become more aware in the present moment. It isn't necessary to sit in the classic meditative pose. Meditation can be performed while lying still, walking, or doing an activity in which you're fully engaged. For instance, contemplative prayer is considered a form of meditation. The goal of meditation is to relate to your experience with a relaxed and compassionate awareness, becoming intimate with the life within and around us.

Meditation can help patients with cancer or other illnesses to better cope with anxiety as well as pain. "On a bodily level, the practices of relaxation and mindfulness reduce the reactivity, fear, and tension that exacerbate discomfort," explains Tara Brach, Ph.D., a psychologist and founder of Insight Meditation in Bethesda, Maryland.

The most familiar form of meditation—in which the person sits comfortably with eyes closed—involves developing concentration by focusing on breathing; repeating a sound or word (known as a mantra); or visualizing certain images, such as a candle flame or a spiritual image.

Another form of meditation, referred to as "mindfulness" or "insight meditation," involves an open and wakeful presence to any phenomenon that arises. You sit quietly, recognizing thoughts, emotions, and sensations, without grasping or resisting the changing flow of experience. Frequently these two styles of practice are combined. With both, the intention is to awaken out of "mental stories": By remaining in the present, with relaxed attention, the heart naturally opens and the mind becomes quiet and clear.

■ HOW IT HELPS ■

Meditation has proven to be so effective in inducing relaxation and reducing stress that it is increasingly recommended by physicians and psychotherapists for stress management; meditation also plays a major role in stress reduction programs for those with serious illnesses.

On an emotional level, meditation reduces anxiety, depression, and stress, which can be of great benefit to cancer patients. Physically, it supports the immune system, reduces pain, and lowers heart and respiration rates and stress hormone levels.

The American Cancer Society's Committee on Alternative and Complementary Therapies acknowledges that meditation can be a helpful form of supportive care. While it doesn't affect the progression or outcome of cancer, according to the committee, it does have measurable—and desirable—physical effects, such as lowering blood pressure and reducing painful muscle tension.

Meditation is often perceived as a solitary practice, but there are many meditation centers that offer group meditations and retreats. Health care practitioners and hospital cancer treatment centers also may incorporate meditation as a part of group sessions. Practicing meditation within a supportive "community" of patients may be especially helpful.

Study after study has shown that patients who practice meditation feel more relaxed and at peace. Apart from the emotional component, patients who practice meditation may experience a marked reduction in symptoms. A study of ninety cancer patients conducted by researchers at Tom Baker Cancer Centre in Calgary, Canada, found that meditation reduced muscle tension, stomach upset, and other stress-related symptoms commonly associated with cancer. The study participants also showed less depression, anxiety, anger, and confusion.[22]

One of the most important potential benefits of meditation for cancer patients is pain reduction. Scientists speculate that meditation may change neural pathways that

MY APPROACH

Tara Brach, Ph.D., is a psychologist and founder of Insight Meditation in Washington, D.C. She has taught meditation around the world and has maintained a psychotherapy practice for more than 20 years.

"Meditation helps people to concentrate, quiet their minds, and find refuge in a genuine inner peace. This allows for the cultivation of mindfulness, a nonjudging, present-centered awareness, and a deep compassion that embraces this life.

"A great area of human suffering is around difficult emotions and obsessive thinking. We either get lost and possessed by the shadow, or we disassociate or disconnect from our inner life. Under this is a deep fear of deficiency and unworthiness. Meditation training allows us to accept and transform these mental and emotional energies through mindful recognition, embodied awareness, and the healing of an open heart.

"The type of meditation that I teach uses the breath and the body as an anchor to reduce distractions and arrive more fully in the present moment. This is combined with mindfulness training (attending to physical sensations, feelings, emotions, thoughts, and consciousness) and heart meditations for loving kindness and compassion. The overall goal is to live fully and love fully, intimate with our inner life, each other, and all beings.

transmit pain; it's also possible that meditation stimulates inhibitory nerves that extend from the spinal cord to the brain. Stimulating these nerves may reduce the sensation of pain.

According to research at the Stress Reduction Clinic at the University of Massachusetts, where meditation is combined with other stress reduction techniques, 65 percent of patients who spent ten weeks in the program reported reductions in pain of 33 percent of more.

■ TRAINING ■

Meditation varies in form and style, and there are many possible sources of instruction, some more "formal" than

---

"My classes begin with instructions and guided meditation to help people relax and be present in the moment. This is followed by a talk on some aspect of spiritual living. It's not religious; rather it offers principles and practical guidance that bring the heart of meditation alive in daily life. Topics might include dealing with difficult emotions, wise communication, the art of relaxation or the experience of fear and shame. After the talk, there is a chance to share observations, ask questions, and hear general announcements about resources in the community.

"Meditation is helpful in addressing physical, emotional, mental, and spiritual levels of pain in those with cancer. Mentally and emotionally, meditation reveals the stories that are distorting and contracting experience. Awareness training allows us to befriend what is difficult, in an honest and kind way. Spiritually, meditation awakens the wisdom and compassion that can most deeply serve our freedom. We open to a sense of intimacy with all life.

"As a clinical psychologist, I regularly coordinate care with a range of conventional therapies. Because of meditation's effectiveness in reducing self-judgment and stress, increasing wakeful presence, and deepening our capacity for intimacy, it naturally enhances a person's receptivity to other healing modalities."

others. It is recommended that you inquire about your practitioner's training and experience and/or observe a class first to see if it meets your needs.

Meditation instruction is not regulated by states; it is unlikely that health insurance would cover it, unless perhaps as part of an organized medical treatment program.

■ TREATMENTS FROM TOP PRACTITIONERS ■

Rudolph Bauer, Ph.D., *is a psychologist, co-director of Washington Center for Consciousness Studies, and director of clinical training at the Gestalt Psychotherapy Training Center in Washington, D.C. Many of his patients have cancer.*

Treatment Goals

Meditation is an ancient and powerful modality for psychological healing and support, says Bauer. It enhances feelings of well-being, awareness, and connection. "In entering the awareness state, people begin to experience a greater sense of spaciousness, lucid clarity, and compassion for themselves and others," he says. "In time, these qualities can become the organizing principle within the personality."

Bauer works with people both individually and in a group setting to teach them to enter and sustain this meditative state of awareness. In his work with cancer patients, he has seen great psychological benefit from meditation.

Treatment Session

Individual counseling sessions last fifty minutes, and are tailored to individual needs. Bauer uses many forms of meditation, including the Dzogchen Tibetan Buddhist tradition, the Hindu Shavite tradition, and the Taoist qi gong traditions. He is also influenced by phenomenology and the work of psychoanalyst Donald Winnicott, which focuses on the necessity of entering into liminal, or transitional, states to facilitate the deepening and expanding of the basic sense of self. "Most of my work centers on entering the naturalistic state of awareness and learning how to sustain that experience," Bauer says.

Benefits to Cancer Patients

According to Bauer, meditation can help cancer patients see themselves as complete individuals, not merely as "patients." "There is often a sense of betrayal by the body, and ill people often live in a state of complete identification with their disease—or in a state of denial," he says. "Meditation helps them enter into an intermediate state between those polarities. Moreover, meditation can assist one in the self-soothing function, which is often so debilitated through invasive medical treatment."

Compatibility with Conventional Treatment

Meditation is very compatible with conventional cancer care. "Meditation is useful in reducing anxiety and helping with the self-soothing, self-regulatory functions," Bauer says. "I work with physicians of many different disciplines, and I also coordinate care with complementary practitioners."

FOR FURTHER INFORMATION

Meditation instruction or classes can often be found through religious or community groups, but the following organizations can provide referrals.

The Naropa University
2130 Arapahoe
Boulder, CO 80302

Phone: (303) 444-0202

www.naropa.edu

The Naropa University, a private, nonprofit liberal arts college characterized by its unique Buddhist educational heritage, will refer people to one of more than one hundred Shambhala Centers throughout the country.

The Insight Meditation Society

Phone: (978)355-4378

A vipassana meditation center, this society can assist individuals in finding a group or instructor in their area.

YOGA

The popularity of yoga in the United States has exploded. Millions of Americans practice yoga, either on their own or in classes offered by yoga studios. One can now even learn yoga at health clubs and local community centers. An increasing number of hospitals have begun incorporating yoga into cancer treatment and other programs, and doctors recommend this ancient Eastern practice because of its many benefits.

Yoga means "union." Its focus is to unite the mind, body, and spirit to achieve a greater sense of well-being, along with better physical and spiritual health. Through its various forms of practice, each of which may emphasize particular goals or techniques, yoga offers the individual opportunities for healing on many different levels. According to Michael Lerner, author of *Choices in Healing*, "the specific relevance of yoga and meditation to cancer patients is clear and profound."

Hatha yoga is the most common form practiced in this country. It originated as part of a health system in India, but it is viewed here primarily as a form of exercise, a spiritual practice, or a combination of the two.

Yoga usually incorporates a combination of exercises, meditation, breathwork (*pranayama*), and postures (*asana*). The postures and exercises can range from gentle to intense, and they progress in levels of difficulty. Nearly everyone, however, can benefit through regular practice of just a few, simple postures.

The breathwork component consists of various breathing exercises that focus on deep, slow, and rhythmic breathing. The goal is to use breath control as a means to physical, emotional, and spiritual release; it also aids in mastery of the different postures. Meditation as part of a yoga practice enhances the benefits of relaxation of mind and body as well.

A typical yoga class involves warm-up poses and breathing exercises, followed by practicing a series of poses that progress in difficulty. Each class usually ends with relaxation poses, breathing, and sometimes meditation.

■ HOW IT HELPS ■

It's hard to think of a condition that can't be improved to some degree by practicing yoga. It's often recommended for those with joint or muscle problems—due to arthritis, for example, or side effects from cancer or cancer treatments—because the postures and exercises increase range of motion, improve alignment, and decrease pain.

Comprehensive cancer care centers, including the renowned Fox Chase Cancer Center in Philadelphia, have created yoga programs to help people recover from the illness—or to better cope with side effects of treatments. Research continues to focus on the therapeutic benefits of maintaining a yoga practice. Yoga has been shown to improve overall fitness, reduce pain, strengthen immunity, and improve circulation, strength, flexibility, and lung capacity.

Harvard researcher Herbert Benson, M.D., who has studied mind-body healing for decades, once observed that Tibetan monks who practiced an advanced form of yoga were able to raise their skin temperature 17 degrees, even while their core body temperatures remained the same. The ability to control body temperature, blood pressure, and other physiological functions with calming exercises such as meditation and prayer has been termed "the relaxation response." Studies have shown that it's a powerful tool for coping with serious illnesses.

Yoga can benefit cancer patients in a number of ways. The breathwork practiced in yoga (one form is known as diaphragmatic breathing) floods tissues throughout the body with energy-giving oxygen, while at the same time lowering the production of stress hormones. This is especially important for cancer patients, who understandably often have high levels of stress hormones, such as cortisol and adrenaline. Over time, elevated levels of these hormones can impair the ability of the immune system to function properly.

Yoga is also an effective way to relieve pain. The practice of yoga, by focusing the mind inward, makes it easier for patients to cope with painful symptoms. The stretching and postures that are an integral component of yoga are among the best ways to release muscular tension, reduce constriction or adhesions of connective tissues, and improve joint lubrication and movement. The physical exercises of yoga promote better circulation of blood and lymphatic fluid.

The emotional benefits of yoga include a higher state of awareness, peace of mind, a sense of calm, and an increased state of relaxation and well-being. "Most clients initially come out of curiosity, but they find that yoga really helps with stress and fatigue," says Helen McVey, a yoga instructor in Arlington, Virginia. "They find that they generally feel better, more supported, and calmer."

Yoga teachers stress the importance of incorporating yoga into daily life, noting that regular practice can induce long-lasting effects for the body, mind, and spirit.

■ TRAINING ■

There are at least six major forms of yoga, each with its own traditions, teacher training programs, and requirements for certification and experience.

Since yoga is considered a spiritual practice and/or form of exercise, the search for a yoga teacher has been considered a personal choice. For this reason many people have been reluctant to create minimum standards for yoga teachers. However, with the recent expansion of yoga into fitness centers, adult education programs, and other nontraditional settings, the problem of assuring teacher competence and experience has become more pertinent. It is recommended that those in search of yoga instruction familiarize themselves with the training and experience of potential teachers.

The recent involvement of health insurance companies has increased pressure for standards to distinguish teachers with solid supervised training and experience from those with minimal uncertified credentials. The Yoga Alliance, an affiliation of yoga organizations and yogis from different traditions, has proposed minimum standards for inclusion in a recently organized national registry of yoga teachers.

■ TREATMENTS FROM TOP PRACTITIONERS ■

Jill Pollet Cahn *is a certified Iyengar yoga instructor in Bethesda, Maryland. She works with cancer patients and others with chronic illnesses.*

Treatment Goals

One of the most important things patients can learn is breath control, which can reduce stress and also improve balance and the functioning of the nervous system. "My second goal is to get my students to recognize and access the energy field," she says. "I love yoga because the poses act as tools to access, clear, and fine-tune the energy field."

Treatment Session

Cahn teaches a variety of yoga classes and workshops, some of which can be quite rigorous. She recommends gentle forms of yoga for cancer patients, depending on their energy levels, side effects they may be experiencing from treatments, and whether they have any other physical limitations or injuries.

"People who come to my Gentle Yoga classes are those who need some support, whether they are dealing with an illness or not," she says. "We start the class by lying down, so everyone is physically supported. Then we move into poses that get the breath and circulation flowing through the body."

MY APPROACH

Helen McVey is a yoga instructor in Sarasota, Florida, who specializes in teaching yoga to breast cancer survivors.

"As a breast cancer survivor, I decided to specialize in yoga for the breast cancer population because of my experience with yoga's impact on the side effects of chemotherapy, and its overall contribution to my general sense of well-being. My purpose in teaching yoga to breast cancer survivors is to help my students find balance and strength in their lives.

"My classes have become a support group of sorts, where a tremendous sense of community can be found. My students are dedicated, interested in, and focused on yoga. They want to get the most from it, so they put a lot into it.

Classes begin with restorative poses that are performed lying down. "The floor work exercises soften muscles and allow us to loosen up and move more easily into other poses," Cahn says. This is followed by midlevel poses—"to get us to lift more effectively from gravity"—and standing poses, which "charge" the body and increase flexibility and strength.

The ninety-minute sessions close with quiet poses, performed while lying down, which are designed to quiet and calm the body. "The poses clear, cleanse, stimulate, and restore," Cahn says. "When you are ill, you need more restorative support than energy output."

Benefits to Cancer Patients

Yoga cleanses the body's organs, improves circulation, supports the immune and lymphatic systems, and strengthens bones, Cahn says. The breathwork taught in yoga assists in keeping the body's chemicals in balance and reduces stress overall.

Restorative poses are extremely important because of their power to boost the immune system, she adds. "The

---

"The emphasis is on accommodating the needs of breast cancer patients. I take into account lymphedema and other conditions or restrictions resulting from cancer treatment, but I still work the students as hard as any Iyengar instructor. Yoga is all about balance, so we strive to find that crucial balance between relaxation and work.

"Yoga boosts the immune system tremendously. Many patients find that yoga helps reduce the nausea from chemotherapy, as well as the stress of daily radiation treatments. It also greatly enhances recovery from surgery.

"I believe that one of the more important benefits is that patients can be themselves in this class. Fear is checked at the door. There is only acceptance and support."

healing power of these poses go beyond the physical realm. They are important during treatment, but also farther on down the line because the healing is so deep."

Compatibility with Conventional Treatment

Because beginning yoga isn't particularly strenuous, and because the sessions can help reduce stress and anxiety, it's a natural complement to conventional cancer therapy. However, Cahn encourages clients to talk to their oncologists or other physicians before starting yoga or other complementary therapies.

■ ■ ■

Patricia Miller *studied yoga in India for nine years, and has been teaching yoga since 1975 in Potomac, Maryland.*

Treatment Goals

Miller teaches Viniyoga, a meditation-oriented form of yoga. "It involves a quieting of the body and mind—a moving away from restlessness and distraction so that we can see more clearly and thus improve the quality of our actions," she says.

Breathing is very important in the approach of Viniyoga, Miller explains. It is synchronized with the yoga positions and practiced separately as rhythmic breathing exercises to calm and strengthen the nervous system. The breath provides the link between the body and the mind. "The emphasis of my teaching is threefold: deepening self-awareness, which includes relaxed, controlled breathing, meditation, and dealing with stress; increasing and balancing muscular strength and flexibility; and building stamina."

Treatment Session

Miller's classes and individual sessions last from one to

two hours. Students begin with breathwork to move into a state that is more relaxed and focused. They work into the practice gradually, beginning with simple stretches. The exercises and breathing techniques are adapted to individual needs.

The first half of the class is devoted to standing poses and sequences of postures that develop flexibility, balance, agility, muscle tone, and stamina. The second half begins with deep relaxation and meditation, lying on the back, and continues with floor exercises that stretch and strengthen the body. The class ends with a breathing exercise that may lead into meditation.

"Most people find that they finish a session feeling a balance of vitality and relaxation," Miller says.

Benefits to Cancer Patients

Yoga is very helpful for stress reduction, and it teaches people how to relax in the midst of tension, Miller says. "It emphasizes stepping back from negative thoughts and letting go of anxiety about results, while encouraging learning to fully experience the present moment. Yoga is effective in helping people cope with pain and the symptoms of serious diseases. It helps people to have more control over their lives and simply feel better physically and mentally. The cancer patients I have worked with have found many benefits from the practice of yoga."

Compatibility with Conventional Treatment

Miller believes yoga is an excellent adjunct to conventional cancer treatments. "The more people relax, and the less stress they experience, the more positively the mind and body can respond to treatments from other modalities," she says.

FOR FURTHER INFORMATION:

The Yoga Alliance Registry may be accessed at www.yogaalliance.org, or (877) YOGA-ALL. The B.K.S. Iyengar Yoga National Association of the United States (IYNAUS) sets standards for certification of Iyengar teachers and has a Certified Teachers International Directory (listing teachers by state) that can be accessed through their web site. Regional yoga networks, community centers, and local health clubs and yoga centers are other viable sources of yoga teacher referrals in your area.

Yoga Alliance
122 West Lancaster Avenue
Reading, PA 19607
(610) 777-7793

QI GONG

Qi gong has long played a prominent role in traditional Chinese medicine. It is a form of exercise that uses controlled breathing, meditation, slow, graceful movements, and focused concentration to direct your "qi," or vital life force.

Like acupuncture, qi gong assumes that good health is dependent upon balanced qi. Qi gong is used by millions of people worldwide to strengthen specific body systems, maintain health, and treat illness. It has been the subject of numerous studies, predominantly in China, where it is a valued and integral part of cancer treatment.

"There's so much documentation in China proving its effectiveness," says Jenny Lamb, a qi gong instructor. "I try to offer patients a different point of view for promoting healing."

Qi gong can be practiced while standing, sitting, or lying down; it can even be done during meditation. It can also be used by healers (qi gong masters), who transmit qi to their patients to help them heal.

■ HOW IT HELPS ■

Qi gong reportedly promotes energy flow, removing any impediments to the flow of life force throughout the body. Benefits seem to include improved organ and tissue function, blood and lymph circulation, and immune system function.

Studies suggest that regular practice of relaxation techniques—not only qi gong, but also meditation, yoga, or even prayer—appears to enhance immune function. Practitioners don't claim that qi gong is a treatment for cancer. But it may help patients with cancer or other serious illnesses ward off infections and maintain a stronger sense of energy and vitality.

On a more immediate level, patients who practice qi gong have reported better pain management. Regular practice of qi gong also appears to lower blood pressure and heart rates; increase relaxation, awareness, and mental clarity; and improve strength, flexibility, and well-being. It is considered useful for many common ailments of cancer patients, such as depression, fatigue, anxiety, insomnia, arthritis, and headaches.

■ TRAINING ■

There is a wide variety of teaching skills and training levels within the practice of qi gong (and tai chi). Many teachers will welcome you as an observer, so it would be worthwhile to visit several teachers, if possible, before you commit to lessons. According to Peggy Li, a teacher of qi gong, "The mark of a good teacher is if they can communicate and explain things well, and if the practice makes you feel better and more relaxed."

■ TREATMENTS FROM TOP PRACTITIONERS ■

Jenny Lamb *is a qi gong instructor.*

Treatment Goals

Qi gong requires considerable self-discipline, according to Lamb. She stresses that people who undertake qi gong need good instructors and the commitment to study and practice regularly. The payoff, however, can be impressive. "I have seen the lives of cancer patients improve through this practice," she says.

The discipline of qi gong brings its own rewards, she adds: "Self-practice is stronger than waiting for someone to help you; healing is always better when it comes from inside." Students often note an increase in energy, better sleep patterns, and less general illness and fatigue.

Treatment Session

Reactions to qi gong vary. Some typical initial responses include feelings of heat or cold, heaviness or lightness, tingling or itchiness. Some patients feel little change initially. Over time, with practice, these reactions subside.

Benefits to Cancer Patients

Lamb has observed "very good benefits" from qi gong for cancer patients. "Qi gong balances the energy sys-

---

MY APPROACH

Shuren Ma is a qi gong master with more than forty years' experience.

"My main goal in teaching qi gong is to enable people to feel their qi. Qi is our life energy, our internal power. It is the essential life force that flows through all living bodies. Qi gong teaches how to connect mind and body in a state of relaxed control, so that you can use your qi for self-healing.

"My basic class consists of a warm-up qi gong exercise for sensitivity; it helps people to feel the qi. This is followed by a standing meditation, which in turn may be followed by a sitting meditation. Sometimes we form healing circles, in which other practitioners and I come together to send our qi to those in need of healing.

tem," she says. "I see improved overall health and strengthening of the body. Stress is reduced. People have more faith and confidence in themselves. They see they can make a difference in their health and have more hope for themselves."

Compatibility with Conventional Treatment

"It would make sense to practice qi gong during conventional cancer treatments because it helps so much emotionally to reduce stress and keep you calm and focused," Lamb says.

In coordinating care, she requires students who are dealing with cancer to notify their physicians when they begin training in qi gong.

FOR FURTHER INFORMATION

The Qi Gong Institute, an organization promoting qi gong through research and education, provides information on research and clinical studies of qi gong. It also provides an international list of member teachers (listed by state) on their web site, www.qigonginstitute.org. Regional networks are a good source of information on finding qi gong instruction

---

"Most people can feel the qi at their first session and eventually even see qi—some describe it as different colors. After a session, they feel more relaxed, more alert, and in a better mood. They are energetic, yet calm at the same time.

"I have worked with many cancer patients, and the improvements in energy, stress, and even skin complexion happen very quickly. I believe qi gong helps improve the immune system, release pain and enhance relaxation of mind and body. People recover faster from illness and injury when practicing qi gong.

"From my work with cancer patients receiving chemotherapy or radiation, it appears that qi gong supports conventional treatments."

as well. Contact local health clubs, community hospitals, community centers, and alternative health organizations for information.

Qi Gong Institute
561 Berkeley Avenue
Menlo Park, CA 94025

TAI CHI

Tai chi is an ancient exercise form popular in China, where it emerged from qi gong hundreds of years ago. It is practiced by people of all ages and fitness levels—which is perhaps one reason for its popularity in the West. As with qi gong, tai chi has become increasingly popular among cancer patients for its ability to reduce stress and tension, increase energy, and improve feelings of confidence and well-being.

This discipline resembles qi gong in that it combines graceful movement, meditation, and breathing to support and direct the flow of qi and attain better health and peace of mind. However, tai chi requires more precision, memorization, and physical space to perform the movements.

Tai chi focuses on maintaining balance, strength, concentration, and calm. It employs a flowing sequence of movements, with one melding into the next. The movements are very slow and measured, with attention focused on diaphragmatic breathing, and are performed in a standing position.

Tai chi is often performed once or twice daily, for about twenty minutes each time. It can be practiced independently or with a partner, and it can be performed anywhere.

■ HOW IT HELPS ■

Tai chi reportedly helps balance qi and strengthen the body; cancer patients often notice improvements in overall flexibility and posture as well as balance, which may help in reducing the risk of falls. The breathing exercises of tai chi impart calm and relaxation. As a form of meditation, tai chi appears to reduce the body's sensitivity to pain and discomfort by reducing stress and muscular tension.

"The basis of our training is raising body awareness and learning how to relax different parts of the body," says Peggy Li, a tai chi instructor. "Cancer patients are soon able to recognize and support their energy. They realize their own power to nourish themselves."

■ TRAINING ■

There are different schools and different systems of tai chi, and tai chi training is often passed from teacher to teacher. Again, there is wide variation in teacher training and approach, and it is advised to observe potential teachers before you commit to lessons. One tai chi instructor I spoke with recommended selecting teachers who have attended professional schools for tai chi training in China.

■ TREATMENTS FROM TOP PRACTITIONERS ■

Peggi Li *is a tai chi instructor in Silver Spring, Maryland. She also incorporates reflexology and shiatsu in her practice.*

Treatment Goals

"In working with cancer patients, my goal is to raise the level of life force to fight the disease," Li says. "We all have an energy system, and we all need ways to nourish that system. These exercises offer the body a healing force that nothing else, including nutrition, surgery, or many other forms of exercise, can provide."

Treatment Sessions

Li offers classes for all levels of tai chi (and qi gong). Each class is suited to different needs and levels of wellness.

The spectrum ranges from movements that are simple and soft to those that are more invigorating and challenging. Classes are usually one hour, and are scheduled once a week for six- to twelve-week sessions.

Patients who are new to tai chi or qi gong sometimes have uncomfortable reactions at first. "Sometimes emotional reactions are experienced, which are considered very beneficial to healing. Physical symptoms can include nausea, dizziness, pain, heat, fatigue, increased elimination, even itchy skin," says Li. "Kicking out bad qi may not be a fun ride."

Actually, most people won't experience these reactions, which can occur with almost any form of natural therapy. They're a common part of the healing process, and are usually short-lived.

Benefits to Cancer Patients

Tai chi increases circulation, which means that more oxygen reaches tissues throughout the body. "This is very helpful for cancer patients, who are typically depleted of oxygen in the area of cancer," Li says. "Breathing is improved, and people also report improved sleep patterns." Li also reports that tai chi is particularly helpful in working out blockages in the upper body and dramatically improving one's flexibility. It's a very effective stress management tool, helping to calm emotions and renew energy.

Compatibility with Conventional Treatment

Tai chi, like qi gong, is completely compatible with chemotherapy, radiation treatments, and other forms of cancer therapy, Li says. "Cancer treatments deplete a lot of energy, and tai chi and qi gong can be very beneficial." Because tai chi is very flexible, it's a simple matter for cancer patients to adjust the sessions according to their time and energy level, to meet their needs at any given time.

FOR FURTHER INFORMATION

Regional networks are most likely your best source of information on finding tai chi instruction. Contact local health clubs, community centers, hospitals, and alternative health organizations for information.

PUBLICATIONS AND TAPES RECOMMENDED BY HEALERS
MEDITATION

Full Catastrophe Living: Using the Wisdom of Your Body and Mind to Face Stress, Pain and Illness. Jon Kabat-Zinn (New York: Delacorte Press, 1990).

The Miracle of Mindfulness: A Manual on Meditation. Thich Nhat Hanh (Boston: Beacon Press, 1996).

A Path with Heart: A Guide Through the Perils and Promises of Spiritual Life. Jack Kornfield (New York: Bantam Books, 1993).

Peace Is Every Step: The Path of Mindfulness in Everyday Life. Thich Nhat Hanh (New York: Bantam Books, 1992).

When Things Fall Apart: Heart Advice for Difficult Times. Pema Chödrön (Boston: Shambhala Publications, 1997).

Wherever You Go, There You Are: Mindfulness Meditation in Everyday Life. Jon Kabat-Zinn. (New York: Hyperion, 1994).

The Complete Guide to Buddhist America. Don Morreale. (Boston: Shambhala Publications, 1998).

Shambhala Sun. Published bimonthly. Reviews, articles, interviews and a directory of meditation, retreat, and contemplative centers. www.shambhalasun.com or at (877)786-1950 or (902) 422-8404.

Inquiring Mind. A reader donation-supported journal, published biannually. Highly regarded for its interviews and articles on Buddhism. Each issue also features an extensive international calendar of vipassana retreats and events, and a listing of sitting groups throughout the country. To obtain a copy, write to Inquiring Mind, P.O. Box 9999, Berkeley, CA 94709.

A number of books on Buddhism and Zen, as well as other topics, are available through Shambhala publications at www.shambhala.com or (888) 424-2329.

MEDITATION TAPES RECOMMENDED BY HEALERS

The Inner Art of Meditation, by Jack Kornfield

The Science of Enlightenment, by Shinzen Young

The Beginner's Guide to Meditation, by Joan Borysenko

Radical Self-Acceptance, by Tara Brach

A good source for tapes is Dharma Seed Tape Library at (800) 969-7333. Guided meditation tapes by Jon Kabat-Zinn are available through his web site, www. mindfulnesstapes.com.

YOGA

The Breathing Book: Good Health and Vitality Through Essential Breathwork. Donna Farhi (New York: Henry Holt and Company, 1996).

Light on Yoga. B.K.S. Iyengar (New York: Schocken Books, 1966).

Relax and Renew: Restful Yoga for Stressful Times. Judith Lasater (Berkeley, California: Rodmell Press, 1995).

The *Yoga Journal* ([510] 841-9200), a bimonthly magazine available in health and book stores, is a good source of information on yoga and other alternative practices.

Living Arts Tapes offers a variety of videotapes for students of yoga, at all levels. Call (800) 254-8464 to request a catalog.

QI GONG

Chi Gong: The Ancient Chinese Way to Health. Paul Dong and Aristide H. Esser (New York: Paragon House, 1990). Contains a chapter on how qi gong works on cancer.

The Way of Qi Gong: The Art and Science of Chinese Energy Healing. **Kenneth S. Cohen (New York: Ballantine Books, 1997).**

TAI CHI

Step-by-Step Tai Chi: The Natural Way to Strength and Health. **Master Lam Kam Chuen (New York: Simon and Schuster, 1994).**

The Way of Harmony: A Guide to Self-Knowledge Through the Arts of Tai Chi Chaun, Hsing I, Pa Kua and Chi Kung. **Howard Reid (New York: Simon and Schuster, 1989).**

Healers also recommend instructional tapes by Kenneth Cohen.

NATUROPATHY

Naturopathy is viewed by many as a gentler approach to health care—one that blends the best approaches of conventional and complementary medicine. It brings together complementary modalities and combines healing techniques long practiced in various countries. While naturopathy employs many of the same conventional diagnostic techniques and scientific technology used by allopathic physicians, there are significant differences in the ways in which conventional and naturopathic doctors are trained, and how each views and treats disease.

Naturopathy, which was formally organized in this country around the turn of the last century, uses only natural methods to strengthen the body's innate ability to heal itself. The body's natural healing responses, such as fever or inflammation, are encouraged rather than suppressed.

Naturopathy focuses on the whole person and not just the physical symptoms. Treatment addresses not only symptom relief, but also strengthens the body's defenses and promotes healing on many different levels. While a limited number of states allow naturopathic physicians to prescribe drugs and perform minor surgery, most physicians do not employ these forms of treatment.

Naturopathic medicine is based on understanding the individual and his or her particular lifestyle, outlook, environment, and other pertinent factors. Practitioners place considerable value on prevention, spending a significant amount of their time educating their patients on health maintenance. Many naturopaths base their practices on nutrition, while specializing in one of the modalities in which they were trained, such as homeopathy or herbal medicine.

Naturopathy can support cancer patients in providing symptom relief, maintaining general health, and making healthy lifestyle changes that promote healing.

■ HOW IT HELPS ■

Naturopathy is not recommended for emergencies or acute, life-threatening illnesses, but can be considered an effective adjunct treatment for cancer when used with conventional treatment. Naturopathy can be helpful in reducing side effects from conventional cancer therapy, and in supporting the immune system and strengthening the body during illness.

"Drugs relieve symptoms, but do not stimulate or encourage healing," says Andrea Sullivan, Ph.D., N.D., a naturopathic physician in Washington, D.C. "I use nontoxic modalities to bring the body back into balance, so that innate processes can stabilize the body and allow it to return to health."

Naturopathy is most successful when used for general health maintenance and disease prevention, and to treat minor illnesses, such as colds and allergies, and chronic conditions, like fatigue and gastrointestinal disorders. Naturopathy recognizes the relationship between emotional health and disease, and has been used to help relieve depression and anxiety, often an issue for people facing chronic illness.

Diet is at the heart of naturopathic medicine, and it's also one of the most effective approaches known for preventing cancer—and for helping the body recover from cancer and cancer treatments. Doctors estimate that the incidence of all cancers could be reduced by at least 30 percent if people would do nothing more than switch to healthier foods.

Naturopaths have traditionally advised patients to eat healthful, balanced diets containing more whole grains, legumes, fruits, and vegetables. But it's only recently that scientists have discovered why plant-based diets are so important.

Consider the following foods, for instance. Studies have shown that broccoli contains a chemical compound called sulforaphane, which appears to prevent normal cells from becoming cancerous. Soy foods contain genistein, a chemical that inhibits tumors by preventing blood vessel formation; and garlic contains allyl sulfides, which appear to destroy potential carcinogens in the body.

Naturopaths often advise cancer patients to eat more whole foods and to reduce their consumption of fats. There are good reasons for this. The fat in animal products and processed foods increases the body's production of free radicals, harmful oxygen molecules that can trigger cancerous changes in healthy cells. Fat also increases levels of bile acid, a digestive fluid that may be transformed in the body into cancer-causing compounds.

For patients who already have cancer—or who are recovering from cancer treatments—the focus of naturopathic treatment moves beyond prevention to relieving discomfort, helping patients cope with their illness and helping their bodies to recover.

For instance, stress and depression can be typical emotions felt by cancer patients during diagnosis, through treatment, and even in recovery. When they aren't kept in check, they can reduce the body's immune defenses, increase levels of fatigue and discouragement, and make it harder to stay positive and motivated. Naturopaths call upon many techniques for relieving these and other "negative" emotions. These techniques include counseling, physical therapy (massage, heat therapy, or manipulation techniques, for example), and exercise, which increases levels of mood-boosting chemicals called endorphins. Patients might be advised to use herbs such as St. John's wort used for depression, or to drink tea made with ginseng, which improves energy. Dietary changes might be recommended as well, because increasing consumption of certain vitamins and minerals can help the body better cope with stress. For example, vitamin B6, which is found in leafy greens, fish, and whole grains, is necessary for the production of serotonin, a brain chemical that regulates mood.

Unlike many complementary systems of care, which may focus on one (or just a few) modalities, naturopathic medicine is extremely broad-based. It's a mistake to think of it as "just" being about herbs or nutrition. Naturopathy addresses the environment, lifestyle, and diet of an individual, and uses many natural therapies to assist a person's own healing resources.

■ WHAT TO EXPECT ■

The first visit with a naturopath usually lasts one hour and involves providing a medical history and undergoing an interview and routine physical exam, along with standard and specialized laboratory work, if needed. During the session, the practitioner will address your specific and immediate health concerns, and will also spend considerable time discussing ways to maintain health and improve your overall lifestyle.

In most cases, patients will be given recommendations for exercise and changes in diet or lifestyle. In addition, patients will be given highly detailed and individualized treatment plans. Naturopaths draw from many different health disciplines; while seeing a naturopath, patients may be treated with nutritional therapy, botanical medicine, traditional Chinese medicine, homeopathy, hydrotherapy, ultrasound, manipulation and other physical therapies, and counseling.

■ TRAINING ■

Naturopathy is increasing in popularity in this country, but there are currently only four accredited member colleges in the United States (Bastyr University, Kenmore, Washington; National College of Naturopathic Medicine, Portland, Oregon; Southwest College of Naturopathic Medicine, Tempe, Arizona; and the University of Bridgeport College of Naturopathic Medicine, Bridgeport, Connecticut). Much of the coursework parallels allopathic medical education, in that students take courses in biochemistry, anatomy, physiology, etc., in addition to specialized training in naturopathic therapeutics. Residency programs, however, are not required. To become a naturopathic physician, a practitioner must graduate from a four-year postgraduate naturopathic medical program approved by the Council on Naturopathic Medical Education and pass state board examinations. There are many naturopathic practitioners who are not physicians. These practitioners have been educated in a variety of training programs and correspondence courses. It is important to interview practitioners to determine their level of training and how they practice their modality, and to be familiar with how naturopathy is practiced in your state. Likewise, as with other complementary modalities, it would be prudent to keep your allopathic physician informed of and involved in your naturopathic care.

Naturopathic medicine is thus far licensed in eleven states. Health insurance coverage varies considerably by state, company, diagnosis, and documentation of claim.

■ TREATMENTS FROM TOP PRACTITIONERS ■

Andrea Sullivan, Ph.D., N.D., *is a naturopathic physician in Washington, D.C., and author of* A Path to Healing: A Guide to Wellness for Body, Mind and Soul.

Treatment Goals

Helping patients to feel empowered and giving them a greater sense of wellness are primary goals of Dr. Sullivan's treatment. "Health includes emotional and spiritual aspects as well as physical well-being," she says. "I have worked with many patients with cancer, and I have noticed that depression from a cancer diagnosis is sometimes more debilitating than the cancer itself. Diet and lifestyle are also very important parts of maintaining health. A large part of my role is to educate patients about their responsibility in achieving good health."

Treatment Session

The first session, which usually lasts ninety minutes, is an exploration of the patient's mental, emotional, and physical health. At the end of the session, Dr. Sullivan gives a homeopathic remedy.

During the second one-hour visit, Dr. Sullivan reviews the patient's diet and provides instructions for following a detoxification diet. Detoxification from harmful toxic build-ups is discussed, as well as the possible use of colonics.

At the third visit, blood type is considered as the criterion for subsequent dietary recommendations. Nutritional supplements, including vitamins and antioxidants as well as herbs, are frequently recommended. Follow-up visits last thirty to forty-five minutes.

Benefits to Cancer Patients

"Naturopathy is very helpful in reducing free-radical oxygen molecules that play a role in the development of cancer," says Dr. Sullivan. "It also helps support the body through chemotherapy, and aids recovery afterward."

"Listening to patients' life issues and allowing them to talk about feelings of depression, anger, and anxiety are equally important," she adds. "Naturopathy helps to educate people on how to become healthier and prevent illness."

Compatibility with Conventional Treatment

Because naturopathy combines conventional and alternative treatments, it's entirely compatible with conventional cancer care. Dr. Sullivan often sees patients who were referred by their regular physicians.

FOR FURTHER INFORMATION

To locate a naturopathic physician in your area who is a graduate of an accredited naturopathic medical school, visit the web site www.naturopathic.org or call the AANP referral line at (866) 538-2267.

American Association of Naturopathic Physicians (AANP)
3201 New Mexico Avenue, N.W.
Suite 350
Washington, D.C. 20016
(202) 895-1392

To learn more about state naturopathic licensing laws and insurance coverage for naturopathy, contact the Alliance for State Licensing of Naturopathic Physicians at www.allianceworkbook.com.

BOOKS RECOMMENDED BY HEALERS

Encyclopedia of Natural Medicine. **Michael T. Murray**
and Joseph E. Pizzorno (Rocklin, California: Prima Publishing, 1991).

A Path to Healing: A Guide to Wellness for Body, Mind and Soul. **Andrea D.**
Sullivan (New York: Doubleday, 1998).

NUTRITIONAL COUNSELING

Nutrition is so necessary for the optimal functioning of the body that it should be a vital component of any healing plan, especially one that involves healing from cancer.

Good nutritional habits help keep the body strong and in balance. They help all of the body's systems, including the immune system, function properly, and they may prevent or reverse conditions that can lead to disease.

But establishing good dietary habits can be hard. Our culturally entrenched poor dietary choices, and the unique needs of each individual, can thwart the best intentions in making nutritional changes. However, because we are responsible for what we feed our bodies, nutrition is one area in which we can make a significant impact on the course of healing. We can make changes on our own terms, at our own pace, and often we can see and feel the results of our efforts.

Individuals can make many changes on their own to establish a healthful diet. Generally considered components of a healthy diet are eliminating caffeine and alcohol; reducing intake of sugar, fat, animal products, and processed foods; eating five or more servings a day of fruits and vegetables; having several servings daily of other plant-source foods such as grains, breads or beans; and drinking six to eight glasses of water a day.

Making nutritional changes as a result of a cancer diagnosis is best done with sound professional advice.

There are many reasons for this. For one thing, conventional cancer treatments can alter nutritional needs and negatively affect the intake, digestion, and absorption of nutrients. Also, science changes rapidly: it seems as though new studies espousing the virtues of the latest "wonder food" or casting doubts on the previously reported benefits of a supplement are always in the media. The very recent past has seen a rapid and far-reaching increase in our knowledge of herbs, foods, and supplements, as well as how they impact on the physiology, chemistry, structural relationships, and functions of the body.

Nutritional science is complex. The mechanistic action of nutrients—amino acids, vitamins, and minerals—can be difficult to understand and apply to your individual needs. Nutritional deficiencies can be subtle and difficult for a layperson to detect. In addition, some nutrients enhance or suppress each other's effectiveness when used in combination. For instance, iron is antagonistic to vitamin E, calcium, and zinc, whereas vitamin C enhances iron absorption. Other nutritional supplements are suspected of interfering with conventional medications or treatments and vice versa. Diuretics, for example, increase the loss of potassium, magnesium, and B vitamins. Tetracycline, an antibiotic, is mutually antagonistic with calcium, iron, magnesium, and zinc.

Even the efficacy and side effects of certain chemotherapeutic agents can be affected by some supplements. Some experts advise against taking antioxidant supplements during chemotherapy or radiation treatments because they are believed to reduce the effectiveness of these therapies. As an example, the American Cancer Society cautions against the use of supplements or foods containing high levels of folic acid when being treated with the chemotherapeutic agent methotrexate, because of its ability to alter the effectiveness of the drug.

High doses of certain supplements may produce harmful side effects. For instance, the fat-soluble vitamins A, E, D, and K are stored in the tissues, which is why high intakes of these vitamins should be monitored with blood work.

Nutritional supplements can be very useful in enhancing the nutrients found in a natural, healthful, balanced diet. They can also be used therapeutically as part of your medical treatment. However, temptation can be great to use supplements for more than their intended purpose. Some people self-medicate with supplements, take larger doses than recommended, or use them to replace medical care. Dealing with cancer can complicate your nutritional needs, and the guidance of a skilled, licensed nutritionist can be invaluable in supporting you through medical treatments, making sound dietary changes, staying current with the science, and motivating you to stay with your new, healthier habits.

■ HOW IT HELPS ■

Scientists now stress the benefits of adopting a healthier diet as a means of preventing disease and maintaining good health. Research on nutrition and cancer provides scientifically supportable guidance on the beneficial role of diet, as well as the virtues of selected foods and nutrients in preventing and fighting cancer and strengthening the immune system.

Nutritional counselors work with cancer patients to develop individualized programs specifically geared to coping with cancer treatment, recovery, prevention, and health maintenance. These programs may include an organic, whole-foods diet; therapeutic, macrobiotic , vegetarian, or vegan diets; fasting and detoxification; juicing, herbal therapies, or supplements; or Ayurvedic nutrition.

"You are treating your cancer for life. The power of nutrition cannot be underestimated in the prevention of illness, in supporting a person through the rigors of chemotherapy and radiation, and in maintaining one's health," says Dana Godbout Laake, a licensed nutritionist in Rockville, Maryland.

The ability of healthful foods to restore immunity—and the power of unhealthful foods to deplete it—is a point worth emphasizing. For cancer prevention, the immune system is the first line of defense: It has the ability to detect and destroy abnormal or cancerous cells before they have a chance to grow or spread. For patients who already have cancer, conventional treatments such as chemotherapy and radiation can significantly weaken the immune system, leaving patients vulnerable to infections.

Cancer patients who see nutritional counselors are often advised to increase their intake of fruits, vegetables, whole grains, and other plant-based foods. Apart from the fact that these foods are rich in essential nutrients, they provide large amounts of antioxidants, chemical compounds that "neutralize" harmful molecules called free radicals in the body. This is important because free radicals damage cells and weaken the immune system.

Eating a healthful diet is just half of the equation; the other half is avoiding unhealthful foods—not always easy. Apart from the fact that foods that are high in fat and sugar appeal to our taste buds, they're nearly ubiquitous in our society. If you go to a restaurant, order fast food, or pick up a frozen dinner at the supermarket, there's a good chance that you're getting a lot more fat in your diet than is healthy.

Obesity is a serious public health issue. According to the American Cancer Society, it is the second leading cause of preventable death in this country, responsible for 300,000 premature deaths annually. It is particularly disturbing to see the significant increase in obesity among children. A high-fat diet is one of the key culprits in weight gain, and excess weight has been linked to an increased risk of cancer. The American Cancer Society has reported that studies have shown a direct association between obesity and certain cancers. Further evidence suggests that obesity increases the risk of at least a half-dozen more.[24] What's more, doctors have estimated a 30 percent reduction in cancer if healthier diets were adopted.

It's not always easy to know which foods are healthful and which are not, which is one more reason why nutritional counseling makes good sense. A nutritional counselor will look at all the foods in the diet. He or she will determine exactly what nutrients you need more of, and which you need to cut back on. You'll also get advice on whether you need to take nutritional supplements.

It's worth noting that many doctors view supplements as unnecessary if you are following a healthful diet. The proper dose of supplements and their use during cancer treatment is also a topic of debate. Some controversy exists about the idea of nutrition as an adjunct cancer treatment. While some physicians argue against the use of supplements, others maintain that the threat of harm from supplements is still largely unproven, and that they indeed may protect normal cells from the damage of conventional cancer treatment. Some nutritional research contains flaws, little supportable evidence, or conflicting reports about efficacy, and new findings in nutrition seem to happen with a high degree of regularity, so there is good reason to be cautious.

Nevertheless, improving nutritional intake clearly helps change a person's internal environment and the conditions in which cancer can take hold and flourish. It can help patients regain their strength and thrive, and improve their quality of life. A healthful, balanced diet appropriate to the individual, along with responsible supplementation, can help create optimal health and well-being, increase energy, improve digestion and absorption of nutrients, support immune system functioning, help prevent chronic disease, and manage stress. And there's solid evidence that certain foods and nutrients can affect tumor growth directly, inhibit tumor-promoting substances, stimulate DNA repair enzymes, strengthen the immune system, and assist in detoxification.

Better nutrition can also speed recovery from medical procedures. It protects against environmental stressors, and helps cleanse and rebuild the body after cancer treatment by reducing the toxic burden and enhancing the body's natural healing abilities. Working with a licensed nutritional professional is the best way to develop an individualized program that is responsive to your particular needs.

■ WHAT TO EXPECT ■

An initial meeting with a licensed nutritionist usually involves providing a detailed medical history, evaluating your current diet, and possibly having laboratory tests to better determine your personal nutritional profile. Some nutritionists are trained to offer a wide array of functional tests that assess nutritional status, food allergies and intolerances, digestion, absorption, and the ability of the liver to detoxify substances.

Nutritional counseling may also include making changes to your diet (including meal planning and food selection and preparation), helping achieve your weight goals, and educating you on supplements, herbs, and other approaches to nutrition. Nutritional deficiencies can be corrected, and reaction-provoking foods avoided, thereby alleviating additional burdens on your body and contributing to improved outcome.

Preliminary dietary recommendations are usually offered during the first visit, and may be adjusted shortly thereafter based on laboratory test results. Follow-up sessions are scheduled to monitor progress and, if necessary, adjust your program. Nutritionists are often available by phone to answer questions as they arise.

It is wise to stay in touch with your nutritionist in order to keep your program current with your needs and with scientific advances. A nutrition program is a process; follow-ups are necessary to fine-tune each person's program according to his or her responses and needs.

It is critically important to keep your physician informed of your diet, any herbs or supplements you take, and any changes you make in these areas. Ideally, your physician and nutritionist should communicate directly, but ultimately it is your responsibility to coordinate your medical and nutritional care to increase your chances for optimal healing.

■ TRAINING ■

The American College of Nutrition offers professional certification through its Certification Board for Nutrition Specialists (CBNS). The CBNS certifies professionals with an advanced degree (masters or doctorate) from a regionally accredited institution in the nutritional sciences (or a relevant field), along with currently licensed medical professionals who have completed additional course work in nutrition. Additional requirements for certification as a certified nutrition specialist include completion of a specified amount of professional experience in the field and an examination offered by the CBNS.

The American Dietetic Association (ADA) has a credentialing agency, the Commission on Dietetic Registration (CDR), for certifying registered dietitians (R.D.) and dietetic technicians registered (D.T.R.). Becoming a registered dietitian requires a bachelor's degree, meeting minimum academic requirements approved by the Commission on Accreditation for Dietetic Education (CADE), completion of a CADE-approved preprofessional internship, and passing the registered dietitian examination, followed by continuing education.

Currently, forty-one states regulate the profession through licensure, certification, or registration. Each state is different and each level of regulation has varying degrees of restriction pertaining to such issues as scope of practice and use of specific professional titles. In states not requiring licensure, persons not certified or registered can still practice. It can be difficult to ascertain the qual-

---

MY APPROACH
Claudia Joy Wingo, R.N., practices nutritional counseling and herbalism at her office in College Park, Maryland.

"My experience as an oncology nurse in Australia has given me a good working knowledge of what cancer clients face, including side effects of treatment. I believe this gives my clients more confidence in my recommendations for herbal and nutritional supplements. I have been straddling the line between conventional and complementary treatments for the past twenty years.

"About fifty percent of my clients are cancer survivors, or have been recently diagnosed with cancer. I specialize in consulting with and supporting those currently facing conventional therapy. I act as a resource guide, providing information and referrals if needed.

"I see cancer as a wake-up call: People need to take a deep look at their lifestyle, diet, environment, relationships, and the ways they view the world. Life changes are not always comfortable to make. I realize that some of my advice is not always easy to follow, but it's vitally important. I believe cancer can be managed, and herbal support can help tremendously.

"I obtain a health history to ascertain the presenting problems, along with a brief personal and family history. I also set objectives with each client, based on needs and current condition. Dietary patterns are

ity of nutritional credentials since so many programs of training are offered and titles vary. Consumers seeking nutrition therapy should be familiar with the qualifications of providers and their state regulations.

In general, health insurance coverage for nutritional counseling is limited to a few conditions.

■ TREATMENTS FROM TOP PRACTITIONERS ■

Dana Godbout Laake is a licensed nutritionist in Rockville, Maryland. Her areas of expertise include therapeutic nutrition, biochemical evaluation, supplementation, and individualized diets.

---

reviewed, along with any current supplements, medications, and recent lab work.

"I make dietary, herbal, and nutritional recommendations. I review general diet guidelines, and also offer several methods to support the immune system, focusing on the Fu Zheng therapy, a form of traditional Chinese herbalism. I'm a proponent of herbal cleansing and detoxification using Western herbs, and I also advise clients on the use of supplements. If appropriate, I'll prepare herbal blends that I formulate specifically for clients and their particular conditions.

"I also touch on lifestyle changes, such as exercise or stress management, and I'll refer clients to other healers as needed.

"Herbs are exceptionally effective for immune support during treatment and recovery. Most clients have far fewer side effects, such as nausea, exhaustion, and hair loss, if they use immune-modulating herbs. They also seem to get back on their feet much more quickly after treatment is over.

"It's important to incorporate herbs and a whole food diet into your regimen over the long term; it's a different way of looking at life. It can be a very enriching growth experience.

"My treatments are compatible with conventional cancer care. Some people don't tolerate some things as well as others, but it is fairly rare when that happens. A bigger issue for me is noncompliance to the dietary, nutritional, and herbal recommendations."

Treatment Goals

"I work with cancer patients to support the immune system, improve their responses to therapy, and optimize outcome," she says. "My goal is to work within their conventional treatment plan. But my work is very individualized. I counsel on everything from a pure vegan diet to a more homogenous plan. The patient determines the level of focus when we first meet, and I work at whatever pace is comfortable for the individual."

Treatment Session

The initial session with Laake lasts ninety minutes to two hours. She takes an extensive medical history and uses cursory nutritional assessment tools to determine the best

---

MY APPROACH

Victoria Wood, M.P.H., R.D., is a registered dietitian and licensed nutritionist who provides nutritional counseling in Takoma Park, Maryland.

"About one-third of my clients are cancer survivors. They are generally highly motivated, educated, self-empowered people who do really well. My goal is to help them attain their goals, which usually include decreasing or eliminating side effects from allopathic treatments, and providing optimal dietary and nutritional support to enhance their immune response and move toward optimal well-being.

"I also want to educate my clients about risk factors for cancer—such as pesticides, certain food additives, chemically produced foods, and chlorinated water—to try to decrease the likelihood of metastases.

"The main focus of the initial session is to give the client very specific recommendations for diet and lifestyle modifications. I work closely with them to develop a program that is relevant and practical. For example, I am very interested in the drugs being used for their cancer because specific nutrients can be used for specific cancer treatments. I provide a nutrition program for them to practice while in treatment, as well as a maintenance program after treatment is completed.

diet for each patient, depending on the type or extent of cancer. Some additional medical tests may be needed for the assessment, and Laake reviews each case with a supervising physician.

During the first session, preliminary supplements are chosen, depending on the condition of the patient's gastrointestinal tract, and whether he or she is currently undergoing chemotherapy or radiation. Nutritional counseling is given at this time and a recommended diet is discussed. Laake is experienced with chemical sensitivities and allergies, and can also advise on detoxification. Later, if the patient has questions about the diet and supplements, Laake is available for phone consultations between appointments.

A follow-up session is usually scheduled within a month,

"I also talk about water, air, and food changes to support the immune system, ways to cook food that are most beneficial to the immune system, and how stress can affect nutrition. In other words, I teach people things that will decrease the load on the immune system, and provide raw materials to strengthen the immune system itself.

"Recommendations aren't always easy to implement, depending on the individual's circumstances and how major the modifications are to diet and way of life. The clients who do best are those who have support, so I try to offer that to them. I am so honored and feel so blessed to be able to participate in the healing process.

"The benefits of nutritional counseling include increased energy, reduced body fat, improved digestion, enhanced immunity, decreased pain, improved memory, possibly fewer medications, a sense of well-being, decreased side effects from some treatments and conditions, and an overall higher quality of life.

"There's no incompatibility between my work and allopathic treatments for cancer. I have worked with oncologists in the past, and am always willing to work with clients' physicians."

so that the person has time to adjust to the diet and supplements. During the one-hour session, test results are reviewed, progress is discussed, and, if necessary, adjustments are made. If the patient is comfortable, Laake schedules a third session in two or three months. She stresses, however, that appointments are based on individual need and can be scheduled sooner if necessary. Once a person finishes cancer treatment, Laake usually schedules a "maintenance session" three to six months later.

Benefits to Cancer Patients
People who are well nourished feel better and have more energy. They're also able to heal more quickly than those who aren't getting all the vital nutrients that they need.

According to Laake, good nutrition is among the most important aspects of cancer care as well as prevention. Cancer patients who have undergone nutritional counseling "feel better and have fewer side effects from chemotherapy," she says.

Compatibility with Conventional Treatment
Some patients may not tolerate supplements while undergoing chemotherapy, but Laake advises that nutritional changes in general are often helpful in supporting the immune system during treatment. Laake is familiar with contraindicators for specific nutrients according to types of cancer and treatment, and can work with a patient's oncology team to coordinate nutritional care with conventional treatments. Laake feels it's very important for patients to work closely with their physicians when making nutritional changes; in fact, she requires that her patients be under the supervision of a primary care physician or oncologist.

■ ■ ■

Irwin J. Rosenberg, P.D. *is a registered pharmacist who has been practicing nutritional pharmacology for twenty-five years. Many of his clients have cancer or are cancer survivors.*

Treatment Goals

Educating people about nutrition is central to Dr. Rosenberg's work with cancer patients. "My goal is to ameliorate or reverse degenerative processes, but it's also important to teach," he says. "I find that if people know what they are doing and why, they are more likely to do it because they alone are responsible for their health."

Treatment Session

Dr. Rosenberg offers an initial counseling session, which lasts for one hour. He gives recommendations for diet, exercise (when possible), and the use of specific nutrients (primarily through supplements) to support the immune system and reduce the side effects of cancer and its treatments.

Clients usually come for one session, returning as necessary when they have questions or particular needs that have to be addressed.

Most clients who follow his nutritional recommendations feel good, but he estimates that about 15 percent will experience a "healing reaction," with nausea or other symptoms that may occur during the body's detoxification process. The discomfort usually resolves itself in three to five days. While the sensations can seem disconcerting, Dr. Rosenberg believes they are a positive sign that the body is purging itself.

Benefits to Cancer Patients

Most clients report reduced side effects from chemotherapy and radiation, and better overall health after the counseling sessions, Dr. Rosenberg says.

Compatibility with Conventional Treatment

Dr. Rosenberg prefers to see clients before they begin conventional therapy, in order to prevent or reduce side effects. But nutritional counseling is also helpful once cancer treatments are under way.

Dr. Rosenberg acknowledges that there is controversy about the use of supplements during conventional cancer treatments. However, he believes that seeking both nutritional counseling and conventional treatment offers cancer clients "the best of both worlds."

FOR MORE INFORMATION

The American College of Nutrition (ACN) offers a referral service for Certified Nutrition Specialists in your area. Contact the ACN at (727) 446-6086. The ACN has a web site, www.am-coll-nutr.org, which can link you to the CBNS.

The ADA also offers a national referral service with a voluntary database of certified practitioners. Visit www.eatright.org or contact the ADA at (312) 899-0040.

The Kushi Institute is devoted to promoting the macrobiotic diet (a balanced diet primarily based on whole grains and vegetables) and a lifestyle more harmonious with nature as a means of preventing cancer and improving life with the disease. The Institute provides referrals to Kushi Institute-trained macrobiotic counselors worldwide. For information, contact the Institute at (800) 975-8744, or access their web site, www.macrobiotics.org.

The American College of Nutrition
300 South Duncan Avenue, Suite 225
Clearwater, FL 33755

The American Dietetic Association
120 South Riverside Plaza, Suite 2000
Chicago, IL 60606

The Kushi Institute
P.O.Box 7
Becket, MA 01223

BOOKS RECOMMENDED BY HEALERS

*Beating Cancer with Nutrition: Clinically Proven and Easy-to-Follow Strategies to
Dramatically Improve Your Quality and Quantity of Life and Chances for a Complete
Remission.* **Patrick Quillin with Noreen Quillin (Tulsa, Oklahoma:
Nutrition Times Press, 1994).**

The Cancer Prevention Diet. **Michio Kushi
(New York: St. Martin's Press, 1993).**

*Prescription for Nutritional Healing: A Practical A-Z Reference to Drug-Free Remedies
Using Vitamins, Minerals, Herbs, and Food Supplements.* **Phyllis A. Balch and
James F. Balch (New York: Avery Penguin Putnam, 2000).**

*Staying Healthy with Nutrition: The Complete Guide to Diet and Nutritional
Medicine.* **Elson M. Haas (Berkeley, California: Celestial Arts, 1992).**

The Chinese approach to diet therapy is a growing field. A recommended resource in this area is:

Healing with Whole Foods: Oriental Traditions and Modern Nutrition. **Paul
Pitchford (Berkeley, California: North Atlantic Books, 1996).**

Healers also recommend works by Dr. Ralph Moss, a science writer
who has spent a significant portion of his career investigating cancer.
You can read about his books on his web site: www.ralphmoss.com. (A
more detailed description of his work can be found in the Appendix.)

People often assume that osteopathy is outside the boundaries of conventional medicine. From its beginnings, however, osteopathy has exemplified integrative medicine, combining allopathic teachings and methods with a holistic approach and unconventional modalities.

Osteopathic medicine was originally developed by an American allopathic physician, Andrew Taylor Still, M.D., in the mid- to late-nineteenth century, who saw the need to treat individuals in a more holistic fashion. The practice of osteopathy is founded on three basic principles: the recognition of the body's own capacity to heal itself, the interrelationship of structure and function in the body, and the treatment of the body as a whole.

Doctors of osteopathy (D.O.s) are fully trained as physicians and surgeons, but undergo additional training in osteopathic techniques. This enables them to provide a multifaceted approach to health care. Many D.O.s practice as general or family practitioners, but may also specialize in any of the recognized medical and surgical specialties, including radiology, surgery, and oncology. They practice in much the same fashion as allopathic physicians in addition to offering complementary treatment options, including manual therapy techniques.

■ HOW IT HELPS ■

One major goal of osteopathy is to improve the structure and functioning of the musculoskeletal system, which is thought to support the body's innate healing abilities.

Osteopathy assumes that disturbances in the musculoskeletal system can affect function throughout the body, thereby affecting how the body works. As a result, many D.O.s give particular attention to the body's mechanics and its interrelationships. When appropriate, the physician may use hands-on treatment to help the body restore normal function.

Because of its focus, osteopathy is a valuable approach for chronic pain, mobility problems, and postsurgical healing. Osteopathic treatment helps to restore normal circulation, nerve function, and muscle and joint activity. It can play a role in nourishing tissues, improving movement, and reducing side effects from cancer or cancer treatments. Patients who have had surgery, for example, may receive osteopathic treatments to increase blood flow, decrease pain, and increase mobility. In addition, osteopathic treatment has been reported to benefit immune system functioning, reduce stress, and improve overall well-being.

Research has shown that osteopathic manipulations can help relieve lower back pain while reducing the need for medications. For those with cancer or other long-term illnesses, for whom imbalances in body posture can result in additional discomfort, this approach may help to improve mobility and reduce pain, with less risk of side effects.

Because of the holistic approach of osteopathy, osteopaths are more likely to place considerable emphasis on nutrition, exercise, stress reduction, and lifestyle issues that can help patients overcome discomfort, impart some control over their illnesses, and have more satisfaction in their daily lives.

■ WHAT TO EXPECT ■

Because osteopaths are trained in conventional medicine, an office visit will include many of the same features as a visit with a mainstream doctor. The osteopath will begin by taking a complete medical history, which is followed by a physical examination, and, if needed, medical tests.

Once a diagnosis is made, the treatments can vary widely. Depending on the condition, patients may be given a prescription for medications or other treatments, along with advice on self-care. Some osteopaths incorporate herbs and supplements in their practices. If appropriate, the doctor may perform an osteopathic treatment at the time of the initial visit.*

The patient lies on an examination table and the physician uses gentle manipulation to lessen any muscular or skeletal restriction, and to restore the body's natural balance and motion. Often the whole body is treated, not just the problem area. Some osteopathic physicians incorporate traditional physical medicine treatments, such as ultrasound or hot packs. More specific mobilizations are sometimes employed as well.

Most people find the treatments very relaxing; treatment effects can result in long-term relief or a reduction in symptoms. In addition to treatment, considerable value is placed on education of the patient, including strategies for prevention. Patients may be taught exercises for better breathing, posture, relaxation, or stress reduction, or receive nutritional advice.

---

* *As with other complementary modalities, in certain situations, such as metastatic cancer, advanced osteoporosis, and certain types of arthritis, direct forms of osteopathic manipulative treatment [OMT] may not be indicated.*

■ TRAINING ■

Medical training for osteopathic physicians is essentially the same as for allopathic physicians. The requirements for a D.O. degree include successful completion of four years of osteopathic medical school, board examinations, and a one-year rotating internship through the primary care areas of medicine. Many choose a residency of two to six years in a specialty area in either a D.O. or M.D. hospital. The American Osteopathic Association (AOA) is the national accrediting organization for osteopathic medicine. There are currently nineteen accredited schools of osteopathic medicine in the United States. Osteopathic physicians' licensing requirements are very similar to those of allopathic physicians and they are fully licensed in every state as physicians and surgeons. They are allowed to dispense the same range of services and are covered by health insurance.

MY APPROACH

Harold Goodman, D.O., is an osteopathic physician who offers homeopathy, osteopathy, acupuncture, and energy healing at his practice in Silver Spring, Maryland.

"I believe that most of what is labeled health care in this country actually concentrates on combating disease. My approach instead concentrates on health. I work to foster and support health in a hands-on, direct fashion. As Andrew Still, the founder of osteopathy, wrote in the 1870s, 'The object of the doctor should be to find health; any fool can find disease.'

"I strive to find those places where proper functioning is impaired because of energy blockages or other causes. I encourage the system with my hands and other methods to restore optimum functioning of the person as a whole. This results in an overall feeling of vitality as well as frequent elimination of many different symptoms, such as pain and fatigue.

■ TREATMENTS FROM TOP PRACTITIONERS ■

Lisa Chun, D.O., *is an osteopathic physician who incorporates cranial osteopathy in her practice in Puhi, Hawaii.*

Treatment Goals

According to Dr. Chun, the physical body can be a reflection of a person's response to both internal and external stressors. "I try to present a forum for optimal functioning and health," she says. "The modality I use supports a person's vitality during and following cancer. It can result in a conscious effect on a person's understanding of his or her true self, thereby contributing to healing."

Treatment Session

Dr. Chun's intake session averages one hour and begins with a traditional medical and surgical history. She also

---

"There is a spirit of health to be found in every cell, in every part of the body. Once the impediments to health have been removed, benefits such as increased energy, decreased symptoms, overall improvement of body functioning, and increased vitality and sense of well-being can be felt almost immediately.

"Cancer touches us where we live. It brings up all kinds of anxiety, fears, doubts, judgments, and other states of mind that block healing. There is a way of going beyond all this: The feeling of peace, and the clarity that comes out of this experience, set the stage for true healing on all levels. I call this spiritual or metaphysical healing. It has nothing to do with a person's religious belief systems, nor is it psychotherapy or an attempt to intellectually understand the emotions. It is probably the most powerful and transformational healing experience I share with patients."

pays particular attention to what many people would consider minor traumas. She conducts an osteopathic palpatory evaluation, and sometimes begins treatment right away, depending on the individual's circumstances. Follow-up sessions are usually thirty minutes long.

Generally, Dr. Chun's patients remain clothed during treatment. She treats most patients lying down on an examination table, but can work on individuals in a standing or sitting position. Her treatment involves an extremely light physical touch to the body. Because cranial manipulation is so gentle, patients' reports range from "feeling nothing" to some warmth or a feeling of release in the body. Dr. Chun also may choose to use active massage and muscle stretching or movement of vertebral segments. As a fully licensed physician, she has the option to use (or suggest) medicines, surgery, and other technical modalities, as well as alternative treatments.

The typical response to her treatments is one of relaxation. Some patients report experiencing fatigue or an exacerbation of presenting systems, but these usually subside within twenty-four hours. Children may have the opposite reaction and become hyperactive following a treatment session, but this also subsides within a few hours.

Rest, water, gentle stretching and breathing exercises, and no overexertion for twenty-four hours are recommended following treatment. Dr. Chun generally likes to see patients weekly for four weeks. Treatment is highly individual; each person is constantly reevaluated based on treatment response. Dr. Chun encourages time between treatments in order to allow for some assimilation. Many patients schedule treatments on an as-needed basis.

Benefits to Cancer Patients

According to Dr. Chun, "abnormal stress can be constructive or destructive. In either case, a heightened physiological response occurs. Prolonged, this can result in physiological and anatomical impairment, not to mention mental, emotional, and physical fatigue."

Osteopathic manipulation addresses these anatomical and physiological changes, strengthening and enhancing the immune system and other related body systems. Her treatment can also help relieve swelling, scarring, poor sleep, or impaired circulation or breathing.

Compatibility with Conventional Therapy

Cranial osteopathy and other osteopathic treatments are compatible with conventional cancer therapy, Dr. Chun says. However, she advises patients to allow twenty-four hours between her treatments and conventional treatment because it takes the body time to adapt to the changes that occur during treatment sessions.

Michael J. Porvaznik, D.O., *is an osteopathic physician and assistant professor of family medicine who maintains a private practice in Arlington, Virginia.*

Treatment Goals

Dr. Porvaznik employs a variety of osteopathic techniques to facilitate healing in his patients. "I help to restore motion in the tissues, the body, and the whole person," he says. "When I use craniosacral techniques, I am actually interfacing energetic medicine with the physical system. I try to be open to patients and listen to what is going on for them without prying. If there are important emotional issues that come up in treatment sessions that a patient does not want to discuss, I refer to a therapist."

While Dr. Porvaznik believes osteopathy offers a lot to

cancer patients, he is open to coordinating care with other modalities. He notes that with his patients, "I am not concerned with *who* gets them well as much as that they *get* well. If problems are chronic and persistent, I sometimes work with other practitioners and integrate the patient's care."

Treatment Session

Dr. Porvaznik's initial evaluation lasts about one hour. It consists of a thorough discussion of the presenting concern, as well as the patient's medical history.

The initial exam consists of a complete evaluation, with the patient standing, sitting, and lying down. Dr. Porvaznik looks for symmetry or asymmetry of bony landmarks, tissue quality and texture, as well as range and quality of motion of the extremities, vertebrae, pelvis, and other areas. He also evaluates the craniosacral system for its quality of motion, which involves assessing the cranial bones, sacrum, dural membranes, cerebrospinal fluid, and central nervous system.

"The osteopathic techniques improve motion and relieve restrictions of movement throughout the body," he says. "They are generally gentle, nonforceful techniques."

Follow-up treatments usually last thirty minutes. There may not be an immediate response to initial treatment, but often improvement comes within one to two sessions.

Benefits to Cancer Patients

Osteopathic manipulation is very helpful for cancer patients because it improves circulation and brings more nutrients to the cells, says Dr. Porvaznik. "It also improves lymphatic circulation, which carries toxic wastes from the cells. There is reduction in pain in areas that were restricted, and also an improved sense of overall well-being."

Osteopathic manipulation is similar to acupuncture in that it helps to restore balance and enables the body to function more efficiently, he adds. "It frees up energy that is being held by tension in the body. People often find that they sleep better, and it's not uncommon for other, seemingly unrelated problems to improve."

Compatibility with Conventional Treatment

Osteopathic manipulation works well with conventional therapies. Dr. Porvaznik often coordinates care with conventional physicians, noting that many of his referrals come from physicians who are aware of osteopathy's unique benefits.

FOR FURTHER INFORMATION

The AOA will direct you to your state osteopathic association to find osteopaths in your area. Contact the AOA at:

The American Osteopathic Association
142 East Ontario Street
Chicago, IL 60611
1(800) 621-1773
www.aoa-net.org

The American Academy of Osteopathy provides a listing of D.O.s, identifying those who use osteopathic manual techniques in their practice. Contact the academy at:

The American Academy of Osteopathy
3500 DePauw Boulevard, Suite 1080
Indianapolis, IN 46268-1136
(317) 879-1881
www.academyofosteopathy.org

The Cranial Academy, a component society of the AAO, provides referrals to physicians with a special focus in cranial osteopathy. (See the discussion on craniosacral therapy in the Bodywork chapter.) You can contact the Academy at:

The Cranial Academy
8202 Clearvista Parkway, Suite 9-D
Indianapolis, IN 46256
(317) 594-0411
www.cranialacademy.org

BOOKS RECOMMENDED BY HEALERS

Dr. Fulford's Touch of Life: The Healing Power of the Natural Life Force. **Robert C. Fulford with Gene Stone (New York: Pocket Books, 1996).**

The Philosophy and Mechanical Principles of Osteopathy. **Andrew Taylor Still (Kansas City, Missouri: Hudson-Kimberly Publishing Co., 1902).**

Philosophy of Osteopathy. **Andrew Taylor Still (Kirksville, Missouri: A.T. Still, 1899).**

Teachings in the Science of Osteopathy. **William Garner Sutherland (Cambridge, Massachusetts: Rudra Press, 1990).**

Those who have lived through cancer often perceive it as a wake-up call, an opportunity for growth or transformation, or a path that leads to a new life. Cancer can trigger the quest for a greater understanding and connection to spirituality: a search for self, for deeper meaning in life, and the profound experience of coming to terms with mortality. I share this view, having found that the spiritual journey initiated by my own illness had a profound impact on the way I healed.

Everyone who experiences cancer faces a basic decision: to find out whether you can embrace the illness as a friend and teacher. One premise I have heard used frequently by healers is that cancer pertains to abundant growth—that cancer is the physical manifestation of this underlying growth energy based in the spirit. Cancer, then, can be interpreted as an opportunity to examine your spirit and find those areas of your life where your growth needs to be expressed.

This growth energy calls each person in an individual way. The opportunities for spiritual growth afforded by cancer require a connection to the basic underlying energy behind the disease. Because this energy is very subtle, most people are not experienced in accessing it and forming a relationship with it. Moreover, its physical manifestation as cancer is threatening to most of us. It can prevent us from seeing cancer in any way other than as "the enemy." But doing so denies you the richest, most vital support you have for your healing: the part of you that's most intimate with your inner growth process.

■ HOW IT HELPS ■

Why do we seek spiritual help? Some choose spiritual direction to assist them in having more meaningful life experiences. So many people I have met have come to me saying, "I know I got my cancer for a reason, and I want to learn as much as I can from it." Others seek blessings from the spiritual realm to help in healing, through rituals, sacraments, laying-on of hands, or soul retrieval work, for example. Spiritual direction can assist in the transition to living with cancer, helping more fully to incorporate the new perspectives and spiritual presence felt during the illness into present, day-to-day living. It can also help prepare for death if necessary, within your own spiritual framework. And spiritual direction can assist in examining spiritual beliefs in the face of cancer and its challenges to your faith.

Spiritual direction can help you find the blessings in cancer. Cancer brings many to a state of immediacy, to living more in the present moment. It can be used as an invitation to enter a spiritual state of creativity *now,* to bring you to be present in a timeless immediacy that accommodates exploration of the vast landscape of the mind, heart, and soul. Cancer is an opportunity to explore your unique relationship with death and self. It is certainly possible to explore the issue and not invite death prematurely; rather, examining the concept of mortality is a key tool for spiritual expansion for many people.

Spiritual direction leads us to our gifts: It can enrich the soul and connect us to the Divine within, our greatest level of inner wisdom. Our life's purpose unfolds through our spiritual work. By gaining a sense of life through the larger context of the soul, we can better understand and

embrace life, come into ourselves with love and acceptance, and live with more meaning, intensity, and integrity.

■ WHAT TO EXPECT ■

While you needn't be well versed in religious doctrine or
feel confident about your ability to pray, seeking spiritual direction or guidance does require something from the
individual. You need to enter this exploration with an
open mind, some courage, a willingness to roll up your
sleeves and "get messy," and a sense of commitment to
the process.

Ann Norfolk, a spiritual counselor, explains that in spiritual work, "one needs a willingness to meet the unknown,
to not understand and yet move forward. Faith and inten-
tionality are vital to the process, even if it is only a willingness to accept help and love. One can start from that."

Your motivation in undertaking spiritual exploration
in the face of cancer is a deeply personal one. There is no
one right way, nor will examining spiritual issues feel
right for everyone. You may feel a clear and powerful call
to spiritual work when facing cancer. The need to seek
spiritual guidance for some is as critical as seeking medical care; for others, those who have never been particularly spiritual, it feels awkward—but they nevertheless
respond to a need to reexamine their life within cancer's
context. They may be trying to define for the first time
their relationship to the Divine, or they may be seeking a
reunion with God or a reconnection to life but are unsure
how to get there.

Many people feel that their only choice is to seek out a
religious leader in their community, revive a dormant religion, or explore a new one. Such a choice can offer famil-
iarity and structure, and lend comfort in the midst of
chaos. But the experience of cancer is often perceived by
some as being so powerful a transformation, and so

outside what they have known, that suddenly religion seems to have no answer for them or seems incapable of bringing any insight. Exploring spiritual issues and cancer within the context of religion may also cause discomfort because of previous negative experiences with religion. Particularly for those who equate spirituality with religion, it can limit or even prevent their exploration simply because they are unaware of other means of seeking spiritual growth.

A distinction can be made, however, between religion and spirituality. Religion usually refers to beliefs and structures—either personal or institutional—that help us express our relationship to God or the Divine. Spirituality helps us find and connect with our spirit, our vital essence, wherever we find our awe, our passion. It can be found through religious traditions and teachings, meditative practices, or some other creative expression such as art, music, or nature.

Spiritual help is not confined to what is provided through traditional religious frameworks. This book introduces you to several alternatives to exploring spirituality and cancer—alternatives that you may have been unaware of, and may be interested in knowing more about. All involve individual guidance, direction, or counseling, and all welcome people of any faith, or no faith at all. What they offer is someone to reflect gently on who you are and how you are choosing to work with the energy of your cancer. The paths to spiritual healing described here are meant to encourage you to try to find the blessings in cancer, and to accept the invitation it holds for wondrous growth, inner peace, and a deepening relationship to self and the Divine through spiritual work.

I would suggest that you be uncompromising in your search for a spiritual director. Each person's training and personal experience is unique and deserves serious consideration. Spiritual work will perhaps be some of the most demanding and rewarding work you will ever do. Finding someone to help you on your spiritual journey is an honor for the individual selected, and a gift to yourself. So choose well. And choose from your heart.

■ TREATMENTS FROM TOP PRACTITIONERS ■

Ann Norfolk *is a spiritual counselor, a teacher at Sevenoaks Pathwork Center, and a pastor at St. James Church in Silver Spring, Maryland.*

Treatment Goals

Norfolk's practice is based on the Pathwork®, which gives a unique understanding of the physical manifestations of spiritual energy. Other practices tend to segregate the physical from the spiritual, but Pathwork helps people gain a deeper understanding of the relationship between body and spirit. She utilizes Pathwork to help patients get to know their core self, and to remove blocks to inner knowledge.

"My goal in working with cancer is to help people have a better relationship with their divine nature and allow for its revelation, both within and outside the context of the disease," Norfolk says. "I want them to get the most possible spiritual identification through their cancer experience, and to help them to know what they are doing, and why, from a spiritual perspective."

Treatment Session

In addition to her Pathwork practice, Norfolk provides pastoral care, which includes sacramental help.

"I see myself as a Sherpa, and the person I am working with as the mountain climber," Norfolk explains. "Even though they choose the path and make the decisions about where we need to go and what we will explore, I know the mountain. I have lived there; I know where the lakes are to drink from, when it will rain and how much, where the steep cliffs are and the kinder short cuts, and how to approach each. I honor the mountain and its gifts, and guide the climber to them."

Sessions usually last one hour, and they may involve talking, spiritual practices, teaching techniques, or energy work.

Norfolk has observed that cancer survivors bring a high degree of motivation to the work. "They have shown a readiness for some inspiring spiritual growth leaps, and I have learned much from them. There is an understanding and appreciation early on of my approach....[T]he energies behind cancer aren't viewed

---

MY APPROACH

Ann Kulp is a staff member of the Spiritual Direction Program at Shalem Institute for Spiritual Formation in Bethesda, Maryland. She provides spiritual counseling and guidance to patients with cancer, or those who are cancer survivors.

"I am a cancer survivor myself. My goal is to be open to whatever comes forth, to be willing to share what is in our hearts, and to allow space for things that are below the surface to come up for exploration, so that we may be honest with feelings and reactions. Through the discernment process, we may uncover different perspectives or achieve greater clarity around core concerns.

"I begin sessions with a lighted candle, and I spend some time in silence with my clients in order to center and become still inwardly. Music may or may not be added as a tool of relaxation. I stress an awareness of the body and what it says to us. We are not disconnected bodies, minds, and spirits. Operating from a sense of the whole, we begin by paying attention to the body and its tightness or tension which affects our openness of mind and heart.

"I rely on clients to bring forth whatever in life they wish to discuss. I have no agenda: It is a trust walk, in a way—to trust in each other and in the work of the Spirit. There is no set pattern for the direction our time will

negatively. I think for many, that is a rare haven for people to come to, where cancer isn't 'the enemy.'"

Benefits to Cancer Patients

"I see having cancer—rather than my work—as a benefit," Norfolk says. "The cancer experience opens people to this spiritual realm, helping to lead them where they need to be. The people I have worked with are more open to living their lives in a more miraculous way. Life is more of a miracle for them; they open to the life-affirming energies and to living the sacred mystery rather than only the 'reality' of our day-to-day existence within the confines of our consciousness and culture."

---

take when together, since we are both—supposedly—awaiting the nudges (or insights or feelings) that arise from attention to the Spirit at work within. During the discussions, I may raise questions for clarification, or there may be pauses for silent reflection. On occasion we may work with dreams or journals, or use sand trays, Tibetan singing bowls, or tangible symbols. It seems to help clients, or "directees," if we explore the areas where they sense the greatest freedom, noticing what helps or hinders that movement. I may comment on what I observe going on, and possibly offer suggestions for ways to pursue identified issues.

"I also recommend that directees spend a small part of their days in meditation or quiet reflection. This can help bring them insight into how the Spirit is at work in their lives, or possibly point to an issue that they wish to bring to their next session.

"I believe that spiritual work helps cancer patients gain perspective, meaning, acceptance, and openness to how this disease plays itself out in their lives, and what good can come from it. It's important for people to allow themselves time, space, and opportunity to get away—to be able to embrace and appreciate the retreat environment, as well as the silence that can bring intuitive knowledge to guide us, and hopefully help us experience a sense of peace."

Compatibility with Conventional Treatment

Norfolk encourages people to seek some form of spiritual direction while dealing with cancer. She is willing to work with physicians, and has done so in the past. "My experience has shown me that many doctors are just waiting for you to take the lead spiritually," she says. "They seem more willing to go through that door with you than you would initially think. Opening that door can led to a much richer relationship with your doctor. I am happy to counsel patients on how to communicate with their physicians on spiritual issues."

■ ■ ■

Gloria Schultz *is a bereavement pastoral specialist and a reiki level II practitioner with a master's degree in theology. In her practice at a Washington, D.C., hospital, she seeks out patients who are currently undergoing—or have already undergone—cancer treatments, providing energy healing, spiritual direction, and guidance.*

Treatment Goals

Schultz says her primary goal is to journey with clients in whatever space they are in, to help them discover that God is with them in the journey.

"My primary work is with cancer patients who are dealing with significant loss," she says. "My goal is to get them to look at their losses, to be with them, and grieve with them. I have a strong sense of the importance of presence, so it's not so much what I say, but the presence I bring in terms of my love relationship with my God that makes a difference."

Treatment Session

Schultz spends most of each session listening and praying with people, being respectful of their religious backgrounds. Her presence is often experienced as very powerful, and her style of prayer extremely helpful. Some people choose to pray with her; others talk or spend the time together in silence.

Schultz conducts healing rounds at the hospital, stopping to work with patients she meets. "I listen to what the person tells me, and then put it in prayer," she says. "I can read between the lines and voice what's been unsaid. This makes them feel really understood and heard."

Schultz concludes sessions by providing feedback and discussing any future needs. "With life issues, I help them to look for options and ways of dealing with them, as I believe that people's answers are inside themselves," she says. "I try to bring them forth."

Benefits to Cancer Patients

It's impossible to underestimate the importance of helping patients to realize that someone truly understands their situation, Schultz says. Healing and reconciliation often occur after a session, along with a deepening sense of who God is. Often, patients are able to find their truth and what they value at a time when they are feeling shattered and broken.

Compatibility with Conventional Treatment

The prayer and counseling Schultz provides are completely compatible with standard medical treatments. Many of her clients, in fact, are referred to her by physicians.

FOR FURTHER INFORMATION

I recommend that you take some time to reflect on Michael Lerner's discussion of spiritual approaches to cancer, found in his book, *Choices in*

Healing. He eloquently presents some of the many facets of spirituality and gives much food for thought to those of us struggling to find meaning in our disease.

One of the forms of spiritual direction described here is through the Pathwork, a spiritual development process based on more than 250 guided lectures on various issues concerning spirituality. For a list of Pathwork Helpers in your area, contact the Pathwork Foundation directly. For kindred groups, follow hotlinks in the Pathwork web site to the Canadian Pathwork site, which has hotlinks to other groups that may be of interest.

The Pathwork Foundation
P.O. Box 6010
Charlottesville, VA 22906-6010
1-800-Pathwork
www.pathwork.org

RETREATS

Retreats are a nurturing rest for the soul and many of us living with cancer find them to be tremendous sources of inspiration, restoration, and renewal. There are many wonderful books listing retreat centers around the country: check your local bookstore and, in particular, religious bookstores. Local churches and synagogues can also be helpful in finding a retreat that's right for you.

And, of course, ask the healers you work with. Many of the meditative practices (yoga, meditation, tai chi, etc.) offer organized retreats that emphasize the body as a means to prayer.

Some retreat programs emphasize silence, which offers a new level of intimacy and connection to the Divine, and can be a tremendous source of emotional and spiritual support. I have found that I schedule retreats and quiet days (silent or otherwise) on a regular basis as a way of loving myself and staying connected to my "soul maintenance."

Finally, many of us gain spiritual insight and a deepening of self simply through our shared experience with others living with cancer. They can be a treasured source of wisdom, leading you to valued information, new ways of thinking and being, and incredible life experiences; they also offer you solace on the journey.

BOOKS RECOMMENDED BY HEALERS

Many beautiful, inspirational books are available for spiritual comfort and insight. There has been tremendous growth in spiritual writing of late; I encourage you to be open to the seemingly limitless possibilities found in contemplative works, poetry, meditation, and other subjects that can be explored at your bookstore or library. Following are some treasures I have found; others have graciously shared offerings from their personal collections.

Care of the Soul. Thomas Moore (New York: Harper Collins, 1992).

Close to the Bone: Life-Threatening Illness and the Search for Meaning. Jean Shinoda Bolen (New York: Scribner, 1996).

A Course in Miracles. (Mill Valley, California: Foundation for Inner Peace, 1999).

Emmanuel's Book. Pat Rodegast and Judith Stanton (New York: Bantam Books, 1989).

Healing Words: The Power of Prayer and the Practice of Medicine. Larry Dossey (San Francisco, California: Harper Collins, 1993).

Illuminata: A Return to Prayer. Marianne Williamson (New York: Riverhead Books, 1995).

The Illuminated Rumi: Translations and Commentary. Coleman Barks and Michael Green (New York: Broadway Books, 1997).

Kitchen Table Wisdom: Stories That Heal. Rachel Naomi Remen (New York: Riverhead Books, 1996).

My Grandfather's Blessings: Stories of Strength, Refuge and Belonging. **Rachel Naomi Remen (New York: Riverhead Books, 2000).**

Now That I Have Cancer I Am Whole: Meditations for Cancer Patients and Those Who Love Them. **John Robert McFarland (Kansas City, Missouri: Nightsong Press, 1997)**

Prayer Is Good Medicine: How to Reap the Healing Benefits of Prayer. **Larry Dossey (San Franciso: Harper Collins, 1996).**

Soul Work: A Field Guide for Spiritual Seekers. **Anne A. Simpkinson and Charles H. Simpkinson (New York: Harper Perennial, 1998).**

The Undefended Self: Living the Pathwork of Spiritual Wholeness. **Susan Thesenga (Madison, Virginia: Pathwork Press, 1994).**

Who Dies? An Investigation of Conscious Living and Conscious Dying. **Steven Levine (Garden City, New York: Anchor Press/Doubleday, 1982).**

For Thou Art With Me: The Healing Power of Psalms. **Samuel Chiel and Henry Dreher (Rodale Books, 2000).**

PROVIDED HERE ARE ADDITIONAL RESOURCES to support your exploration and selection of complementary modalities and healers. Included here are listings of books of a more general nature, journals and sources for audiotapes, and organizations providing information, support, wellness programs, treatments, and referrals. Please review the "For Further Information" and "Books Recommended by Healers" sections of each Modality description for additional recommendations on books and organizations.

The world of resources for complementary and alternative therapies is continually enriched with new research, treatments, programs, and information. To enrich yourself, you will need to stay current. I encourage you to check in with your local bookstore, peruse the literature from time to time, and visit the Internet when you feel the need. And don't forget your network of survivors and healers. Keep passing it on.

BOOKS

General Reference

The Alternative Medicine Handbook: The Complete Guide to Alternative and Complementary Therapies. Barrie Cassileth, Ph.D. (New York: W.W. Norton and Company, 1998).

Alternative Medicine: The Definitive Guide. Compiled by The Burton Goldberg Group (Fife, Washington: Future Medicine Publishing Group, 1993)_

Alternative Medicine: What Works: A Comprehensive, Easy-to-Read Review of The Scientific Evidence, Pro and Con. Adriane Fugh-Berman (Baltimore: Lippincott, Williams & Wilkins, 1997).

American Cancer Society's Guide to Complementary and Alternative Cancer Methods. Atlanta: The American Cancer Society. Available in bookstores and on-line: www.cancer.org or (888) 227-5552.

The Best Alternative Medicine: What Works? What Does Not? Kenneth Pelletier, M.D. (New York: Simon and Schuster, 2000)

Beyond Miracles: Living With Cancer: Inspirational and Practical Advice for Patients and Their Families. Steven P. Hersh (Lincolnwood, Illinois, Seven Locks Press, 2000).

Cancer and Natural Medicine: A Textbook of Basic Science and Clinical Research. John Boik (Princeton, Minnesota: Oregon Medical Press, 1995).

Cancer Therapy: The Independent Consumer's Guide to Non-Toxic Treatment and Prevention. Ralph W. Moss (New York, New York: Equinox Press, 1993).

Choices in Healing: Integrating the Best of Conventional and Complementary Approaches to Cancer. Michael Lerner (Cambridge, Massachusetts: The MIT Press, 1994). Can be found on-line in its entirety: www.commonweal.org/choicescontents.html.

Comprehensive Cancer Care: Integrating Alternative, Complementary, and Conventional Therapies. James S. Gordon and Sharon Curtin (Cambridge, Massachusetts: Perseus Publishing, 2000). This book provides an excellent and insightful guide to accessing the Internet and descriptions of web site resources.

Essentials of Complementary and Alternative Medicine. Wayne B. Jonas and Jeffrey S. Levin, eds. (Baltimore: Lippincott, Williams and Wilkins, 1999).

First Aid Yourself: Essential Breast Cancer Websites. Betsy Dance (Manakin-Sabot, Virginia: Hope Springs Press, Inc., 2000). An excellent source of web sites, many of which are appropriate for other cancers as well. Selected pages of the book are available on-line: www.firstaidyourself.org.

Manifesto for a New Medicine: Your Guide to Healing Partnerships and the Wise Use of Alternative Therapies. James S. Gordon (Reading, Massachusetts: Addison-Wesley Publishing Co., 1996).

Options: The Alternative Cancer Therapy Book. Richard Walters (Garden City Park, New York: Avery Penguin Putnam, 1992).

Third Opinion: An International Directory to Alternative Therapy Centers for the Treatment of Cancer and Other Degenerative Diseases. John Fink (Garden City Park, New York: Avery Penguin Putnam, 1992).

Integrative Healing

Cancer as a Turning Point: A Handbook for People with Cancer, Their Families and Health Professionals. Lawrence LeShan (New York: Plume Publishing, 1999).

The Journey Through Cancer: An Oncologist's Seven-Level Program for Healing and Transforming the Whole Person. Jeremy R. Geffen (New York: Crown Publishers, 2000).

Love, Medicine and Miracles: Lessons Learned About Self-Healing from a Surgeon's Experience With Exceptional Patients. Bernie Siegel (New York: Harper Collins, 1986).

Mind-Body

The Immune Power Personality: 7 Traits You Can Develop to Stay Healthy. Henry Dreher (New York: Dutton, 1995).

Molecules of Emotion: The Science Behind Mind-Body Medicine. Candace B. Pert (New York: Simon and Schuster, 1997).

Timeless Healing: The Power and Biology of Belief. Herbert Benson (New York: Fireside, 1997).

Treatment Planning

Self-Healing Journal: Collections, Explorations and Learnings for My Personal Health Journey. Betty A. Caldwell and Georgia D. Dow (Columbia, Maryland: Healing Dimensions Foundation, 1999.) This personalized journal is a useful way to record the development of your own integrative treatment plan. Order through the Healing Dimensions Foundation: (410)740-4659.

JOURNALS

Alternative and Complementary Therapies
(800) 654-3237
www.liebertpub.com/act
Official journal of the Society of Integrative Medicine. Bimonthly publication for health care practitioners.

Alternative Medicine Review
(800) 228-1966
www.thorne.com.
Reviews of current scientific research on alternative therapies.

Alternative Therapies in Health and Medicine
(866) 828-2962
www.alternative–therapies.com.
Published bimonthly; mind-body emphasis.

Integrative Cancer Therapies
(800) 818-7243
www.sagepub.co.uk.
Quarterly journal geared toward clinicians and health care professionals

Journal of Alternative and Complementary Medicine
(800) 654-3237
Articles on clinical research; published bimonthly.

TAPES

Simonton Cancer Center
(800) 338-2360
www.simontoncenter.com.
Audiotapes on attitudinal work, affirmations, guided imagery, meditation, relaxation and specific health conditions.

Sounds True
(800) 333-9185
www.soundstrue.com.
Audiotapes on such subjects as meditation, psychology, spirituality, and creativity.

Health Journeys

(800) 800-8661

www.healthjourneys.com

Audiotapes and CDs on various topics, including affirmations, cancer, chemotherapy, depression, general wellness, healthful sleep, pain, radiation therapy, and stress. Many of the guided imagery audiotapes and CDs feature Belleruth Naparstek. Other tapes available for adults and children on selected topics.

Exceptional Cancer Patients

(814) 337-8192

www.ecap-online.org.

Wellness-oriented videotapes, audiotapes and books; includes works by Bernie Siegel, M.D., founder.

Hay House

(800) 654-5126

Self-help and inspirational tapes.

ORGANIZATIONS

Alternative Medicine Foundation

P.O. Box 60016

Potomac, MD 20859

(301) 340-1960/public information inquiries (voice mail only):

www.amfoundation.org

Non-profit organization providing information to the public regarding the integration of alternative and conventional medicine. Has comprehensive website that includes information on choosing practitioners, referral services for holistic practitioners, and resource guides on selected complementary modalities and health issues, including cancer.

American College for Advancement in Medicine

23121 Verdugo Drive, Suite 204

Laguna Hills, CA 92653

www.acam.org

Medical society providing information on alternative and complementary therapies appropriate to cancer. Provides referrals to approximately 1,000 member physicians. Focus on chelation therapy in physician training programs.

American Holistic Health Association
P.O.Box 17400
Anaheim, CA 92817-7400
(714) 779-6152
www.ahha.org

Web site includes a database of over 200 AHHA members who practice holistic health care and represent a range of modalities; over 60 referral sources to additional practitioners; a listing of AHHA institutional members who provide integrative health care or alternative therapies; a listing of organizations providing health information search services, and other resources.

American Holistic Medical Association
12101 Menaul Boulevard, N.E.
Suite C
Albuquerque, NM 87112
(505) 292-7788
www.holisticmedicine.org

The AHMA provides a referral directory of their members, which include licensed M.D.s and D.O.s practicing holistic medicine, along with medical students, residents and interns. The web site also contains information on cancer-related complementary/alternative therapies and selecting holistic practitioners.

Block Medical Center/Institute for Integrative Cancer Care
1800 Sherman Avenue, Suite 515
Evanston, IL 60201
(847) 492-3040
www.blockmd.com

The Block Medical Center and the Institute for Integrative Cancer Care combines conventional medicine with cutting-edge complementary therapies for an individualized approach to cancer treatment. Services include chronotherapy (circadian timing to reduce drug toxicity and improve results), personalized nutrition, supplement and herbal strategies, and patient education.

Cancer Treatment Centers of America
(800) 615-3055/(800) 234-0497
www.cancercenter.com

Holistic treatment program offered in several locations in the United States, providing traditional cancer therapies in combination with mind/body approaches, nutrition and naturopathic, psychological and spiritual support. Web site has searchable database that includes comparisons of conventional and alternative cancer treatments.

CanHelp
3111 Paradise Bay Road
Port Ludlow, WA 98365
(800) 565-1732/ (360) 437-2291
www.canhelp.com

Information and referral service for cancer patients. For a fee ($400-$550), will analyze individual's medical records, conduct a search of alternative and conventional treatments, and confer with both traditional and alternative medical experts to produce an individualized report of appropriate treatment options and provider referrals. Directed by Patrick McGrady, medical writer, author and advocate for cancer patients' rights.

Center for Mind Body Medicine
5225 Connecticut Avenue, N.W., Suite 414
Washington, D.C. 20015
(202) 966-7338
www.cmbm.org

CMBM works toward creating transformational healing models and facilitating their availability and accessibility. The Center offers instruction in mind-body skills via support groups for people with cancer and other conditions, a volunteer physician CancerGuide to help people evaluate therapeutic options, and professional training programs, and hosts an annual conference on complementary cancer care. The Center has recently created a training program for CancerGuides—integrative care counselors for people with cancer and their families. A national directory of resources, organizations, and practitioners of complementary care is available through the Center.

Commonweal
P.O. Box 316
Bolinas, CA 94924
(415) 868-0970
www.commonweal.org

The Commonweal Cancer Help Program offers small group week-long retreats for individuals with cancer, supporting them spiritually and emotionally in their exploration of healing. Commonweal provides a free telephone referral service of practitioners, treatments and clinics that past participants of the Commonweal Cancer Help Program (primarily from the East and West coasts) wish to share with other cancer patients. Referrals often include the name and telephone number of the referring patient. To access the CanServe database, call Mimi Mindel at Commonweal.

Exceptional Cancer Patients
522 Jackson Park Drive
Meadville, PA 16335
(814) 337-8192
www.ecap-online.org

ECaP, founded by Bernie Siegel, M.D., offers cancer patients retreats, seminars, programs, materials, and information to support the healing of body, mind, and spirit from cancer. (There are also training programs offered for health care professionals.) ECaP offers a listing of members (practitioners who have participated in ECaP workshops), listed by their licensed practice state and what services they provide. The web site also lists wellness-oriented videos, books, and tapes by Dr. Siegel and other authors.

Geffen Cancer Center and Research Institute
981 37th Place
Vero Beach, FL 32960
(800) 834-4791 or (772) 770-5800
www.geffencenter.com

Integrative center offering conventional treatment in combination with nutrition, counseling, massage, meditative practices, acupuncture and other complementary therapies. The web site contains information on Dr. Geffen's Seven-Level Cancer Program, and offers a recommended list of books, audiotapes, and CDs.

The Gerson Institute
1572 Second Avenue
San Diego, CA 92101
(888)-4-GERSON
(619) 685-5353
www.gerson.org

Provides holistic therapy (primarily dietary treatment and detoxification) for degenerative diseases, including cancer. Web site describes therapy and treatment centers.

Healing Choices/Cancer Chronicles
The Moss Reports
P.O. Box 1076
Lemont, PA 16851
(800) 980-1234
www.ralphmoss.com, www.cancerdecisions.com

Offers detailed reports on treatment options specific to particular cancer diagnoses prepared by Ralph Moss, Ph.D., author of numerous books on cancer. The "Moss Reports" discuss both appropriate conventional treatments, innovative therapies and alternative/complementary therapies and how to get them. The cost of a treatment report is approximately $300, and includes follow-up consultations.

Health Resources, Inc.
933 Faulkner
Conway, AZ 72032
(800) 949-0090
(501) 329-5272
www.thehealthresource.com

Medical information service provides individualized reports of available conventional and alternative/complementary therapies for specific types of cancer. Current cost is $395 plus shipping charges.

National Center for Complementary and Alternative
Medicine (NCCAM) Clearinghouse
P.O. Box 7923
Gaithersburg, MD 20898
(888) 644-6226
http://nccam.nih.gov

The National Center for Complementary and Alternative Medicine of the National Institutes of Health conducts and supports research to evaluate alternative and complementary therapies. The clearinghouse provides information to practitioners and the public on research regarding alternative and complementary treatments.

National Foundation for Alternative Medicine
1629 K Street, N.W., Suite 402
Washington, D.C. 20006
(202) 463-4900
www.nfam.org

Detailed information on more than 50 alternative cancer clinics–primarily abroad–visited and investigated by NFAM. Information on several clinics is available on the NFAM web site; otherwise, information is provided in response to a telephone or written request at no charge.

Omega Institute of Holistic Studies
150 Lake Drive
Rhinebeck, NY 12572
(800) 944-1001 or (845) 266-4444
www.eomega.org

The Institute hosts workshops, spiritual retreats, and wellness programs on a variety of topics, including music, dance and movement, yoga, qi gong and martial arts, spiritual practice, shamanism, and creative expression.

Simonton Cancer Center
P.O. Box 890
Pacific Palisades, CA 90272
(800) 459-3424
www.simontoncenter.com

Five-day program offering psychotherapeutic support and education to cancer patients and their spouses or supporters.

Sun Farm Corporation
P.O. Box 5272
Milford, CT 06460
(203) 882-8000
www.sunfarmcorp.com.

Sun Farm Corporation, founded by Dr. Alexander Sun, a biochemist, produces Sun Farm Vegetable Soup, a food supplement that shows promise for use in cancer treatment. (I have incorporated the soup into my nutritional program since my own diagnosis, and continue to follow its progress.) Several clinical trials have been completed on the soup, which contains natural ingredients known to have anti-tumor or immune-enhancing components. For further information on the soup and research results, visit their web site.

University of Massachusetts Memorial Health Center
Stress Reduction Clinic/Center for Mindfulness
55 Lake Avenue, North
Worcester, MA 01655
(508) 856-2656
www.umassmed.edu/cfm/srp.

Offers eight-week courses on mindfulness meditation, yoga, pain management, and stress management, based on the work of Jon Kabat-Zinn.

The Wellness Community
35 East 7th Street, Suite 412
Cincinnati, OH 45202
(888) 793-9355 (WELL)
www.thewellnesscommunity.org

Extensive network of psychosocial support for individuals and families dealing with cancer. Offers non-residential support groups, educational workshops, stress management programs, and other services free of charge at facilities in various locations throughout the United States.

World Research Foundation
41 Bell Rock Plaza
Sedona, AZ 86351
(928) 284-3300
www.wrf.org

Medical research foundation provides information on therapies and treatment options (both conventional and alternative/complementary) and referral information for cancer patients.

WEB SITES

The following selection of web sites may be of interest to the reader. There are many more excellent web sites available that are relevant to researching integrative cancer care or that offer support to cancer survivors, some of which are included earlier in the Appendix or in the Modality Descriptions.

CancerNet-Complementary and Alternative Medicine
http://www.cancer.gov/cancerinfo/treatment/cam
Scientific information on complementary and alternative cancer treatments from the National Cancer Institute. Provides information on treatment options, clinical trials, and other topics of interest to cancer patients.

CANSearch: Guide to Cancer Resources on the Internet
www.canceradvocacy.org
   The National Coalition for Cancer Survivorship guide to on-line cancer resources.

Heal USA
www.healusa.net
   Promotes the reponsible use of integrative medicine by providing a Medical Standards Program for qualified alternative practitioners. Provides a weekly e-mail newsletter on alternative treatments, guidelines on credentialing, and quality assurance standards. Videos on survivors' use of integrative medicine.

Health World Online
www.healthy.net
   Expansive web site covers a vast array of topics from descriptions on alternative treatments and advice on finding practitioners to integrative cancer care. Contains a referral network of holistic practitioners, based on professional organization membership.

Medline/PubMed
http://www.ncbi.nlm.nih.gov/entrez/query.fcgi
   A free service of the National Library of Medicine, offering access to medical journals and over 12 million Medline citations.

OncoLink

www.oncolink.com

Oncology information resource from the University of Pennsylvania Cancer Center. Contains information on current research in cancer treatments, mostly conventional, and on a variety of topics, including global resources, symptom management, and coping with cancer. Contains write-ups of selected complementary therapies and their applications to cancer. The site offers a recommended reading list for complementary medicine, with book reviews.

Rosenthal Center for Complementary and Alternative Medicine

http://www.rosenthal.hs.columbia.edu

Information and comprehensive listing of on-line resources on alternative and complementary medicine modalities for cancer.

Steve Dunn's CancerGuide

www.cancerguide.org

Information on cancer and guide to researching cancer, clinical trials, understanding statistics, evaluating alternative treatments, research resources for alternative cancer therapies and other topics provided by cancer survivor Steve Dunn.

REFERENCES

1. Richardson, MA, et al. Complementary/alternative use in a comprehensive cancer center and the implications for oncology. *Journal of Clinical Oncology* 18: 2505–2514, 2000.

2. Galland, Leo. *The Four Pillars of Healing: How the New Integrated Medicine Can Cure You* (New York: Random House, 1997), pp. 1-20.

3. Gordon, James M. *Manifesto for a New Medicine: Your Guide to Healing Partnerships and the Wise Use of Alternative Therapies* (New York: Addison-Wesley, 1996), p. 110.

4. Speigel, David, et al. Effect of psychosocial treatment on survival of patients with metastatic breast cancer. *Lancet* II (8668), pp. 888-891, October 14, 1989.

5. Lazarou, Jason, et al. Incidence of adverse drug reactions in hospitalized patients. *Journal of the American Medical Association* 279: 1200-1205, April 15, 1998.

6. Boon, Heather, et al. Use of complementary/alternative medicine by breast cancer survivors in Ontario: prevalence and perceptions. *Journal of Clinical Oncology* 18: 2515–2521, 2000.

7. Adler, S.R., and Fosket, J.R., as cited in Integrating complementary medicine into cancer care. *The Oncology Roundtable*, 19: p. 2, 2000.

8. Burstein, Harold J. Discussing complementary therapies with cancer patients: what should we be talking about? *Journal of Clinical Oncology*, 18: 2501-2503, 2000.

9. Shen, J., Wenger, N., Glaspy, J., et al. Electroacupuncture for control of myeloablative chemotherapy–induced emesis: a randomized controlled trial. *Journal of the American Medical Association*, 284:2755–2761, 2000.

10. Ferrell-Terry, A.T., and Glick, O.J. The use of therapeutic massage as a nursing intervention to modify anxiety and the perception of cancer pain. *Cancer Nursing*, 16:93–101, 1993.

11. Wilkie, D.J., Kampbell J., Cutshall, S., et al. Effects of massage on pain intensity, analgesics, and quality of life in patients with cancer pain: a pilot study of a randomized clinical trial conducted within hospice care delivery. *The Hospice Journal*, 15:31–51, 2000.

12. Zeitlin, Diane, et al. Unpublished study funded by the American Massage Therapy Association.

13. Hernandez-Reif, M., Field, T., Ironson, G., Weiss, S., and Katz, G. Immunological responses of breast cancer patients to massage therapy. Manuscript in review, March 2002.

14. Dibble, S.L., Chapman, J., Mack, K.A., and Shih, A.S. Acupressure for nausea: results of a pilot study. *Oncology Nursing Forum*, 27:41–47, 2000.

15. Schneider, J., Gilford, S. The chiropractor's role in pain management for oncology patients. *Journal of Manipulative and Physiological Therapeutics*, 24:52–57, 2001.

16. Gruber, B., et al. Immunological responses of breast cancer patients to behavioral interventions. *Biofeedback and Self-Regulation*, 18:1-22, 1993.

17. Gruber, B., et al. Immune system and psychological changes in metastatic cancer patients while using ritualized, relaxation and guided imagery. *Scandinavian Journal of Behavior Therapy*, 17:25–46, 1988.

18. Syrjala, K.L., Donaldson G. W., Davis, M.W., Kippes M.E., and Carr, J.E. Relaxation and imagery and cognitive-behavioral

training reduce pain during cancer treatment: a controlled clinical trial. *Pain*, 63:189–198, 1995.

19. Tusek, D., Church, J.M., and Fazio, V.W. Guided imagery as a coping strategy for perioperative patients. *Association of Operating Room Nurses Journal*, 66:644–649, 1997.

20. Kleijnen, J., Knipschild, P., and Rieter, G. Clinical trials of homeopathy. *British Medical Journal*, 302:316–323, 1991.

21. Balzarini, A., Felisi, E., Martini, A., and DeConno, F. Efficacy of homeopathic treatment of skin reactions during radiotherapy for breast cancer: a randomised, double-blind clinical trial. *British Homeopathy Journal*, 89:8–12, 2000.

22. Speca, M., Carlson, L.E., Goodey, E., and Angen, M. A randomized, wait-list controlled clinical trial: the effect of a mindfulness meditation-based stress reduction program on mood and symptoms of stress in cancer outpatients. *Psychosomatic Medicine*, 62:613–622, 2000.

23. American Cancer Society. *Cancer Facts and Figures, 2001*. Atlanta, Georgia: ACS, 2001.

THIS IS A SPECIAL PLACE for you to record your answers to the exercises contained in the book and your experiences in developing your own integrated treatment plan. I encourage you to record as much of your healing as you wish, for several reasons. Having a written record of your complementary treatment decisions will help you in coordinating your care with your physicians and other health professionals. But just as importantly, it is a rich journey you are embarking upon, and returning to these pages from time to time may comfort and inspire you and perhaps others with whom you might share your wisdom and insight.